DETERMINATION

Also Written By

Sarah Todd Hammer and Jennifer Starzec:

5k, Ballet, and a Spinal Cord Injury

DETERMINATION

Sarah Todd Hammer   **Jennifer Starzec**

Printed in the United States of America

Hammer, Sarah Todd; Starzec, Jennifer.

Determination / Sarah Todd Hammer ; with Jennifer Starzec

This book is about true events. However, some people's names have been changed to protect

their identity.

Some events may not be exactly as they happened in real life. The events are as the authors

remember them.

4

Dedicated To

My great Aunt Joan and Uncle John. I know you are as

determined as ever.

- Sarah Todd

My Mima and Beepa. I miss you a ton.

- Jen

Table of Contents

With my hair in a long, beautiful braid
And lips shimmering from bright, pink gloss,
I hoped my dance would get my point across.
Though I could not help but feel quite afraid,
When I started to dance, all my fears strayed.
The stage eliminated all things dross—
And, although dancing and prancing exhausts,
I was proud of the memory I made.

Cheers, yells, and screams greeted my smiling face,
Running off the stage and hugging my friend.
Tears collected, falling, dripping, around;
I knew this ended my successful race.
The experience helped many hearts mend—
There, happiness had started to abound.

Poem by Sarah Todd Hammer

Courage.

Sarah Todd

I stood in the bathroom at the Center For Courageous Kids, waiting patiently while Jen did my makeup for my dance "Adrift," which I was getting ready to perform in the camp talent show.

"Oops! I didn't mean to get mascara there!" Jen exclaimed. I giggled as she rushed to her room (that connected to mine, oh so conveniently), to grab a Q-tip to wash off the unwanted mascara that was just below my eyes. She quickly returned and scrubbed it off before reaching into my new makeup bag to grab my sparkly-white eyeshadow.

"There!" Jen stepped back, looking over my makeup she had done, to make sure it was up to par. Relieved she was finished (I had been standing for a long time), I stole a quick glance in the mirror, pleased with the way everything looked.

We made our way down to the dining hall where the stage was and where the talent show would be held. Jen and I went over to the restrooms to make sure my costume—which was a beautiful gray and white dress with sequins—and that my hair, which was done up in a messy side-braid, looked acceptable. After checking everything, we strode to the back of the audience and looked through the program to see when I would be on. We learned that I was the sixth act, and we had to be backstage three acts before my own. So, I tried to relax, seeing as I was becoming slightly nervous, and drank some water so I'd be hydrated and full of energy for the dance. When the second act was over, Jen and I scurried backstage, eager to get the show on the road. While we waited, I ran through the dance in my head, making sure I wouldn't forget it.

"Jen, what do I do after the chorus?!" I said worriedly, thinking I didn't know my dance, which I had choreographed myself. I could tell it was just the nerves getting to me—I knew that in the back of my mind—I just didn't want to end up having to improvise in front of an audience.

"Don't worry, once you start it, you'll remember it all," she reassured me. I knew she was right, and I also knew that I remembered my whole dance from beginning to end. She then helped me slip on my ballet shoes, which were just traditional slippers, so I'd be ready on time.

The line of people waiting was moving forward little by little, and soon, I was watching the fifth act from behind the curtain. When the little girl was done singing "Let It Go" from the Disney movie *Frozen*, it was my turn to perform.

Jen sat in a chair backstage, her iPhone ready to record the whole thing. A few people were recording it from the audience, too.

The announcer's voice bellowed through the rather large room, saying, "next we have Sarah Todd, performing her dance, 'Adrift!'" The crowd cheered and clapped, and I gave Jen a quick hug, before walking a bit onto the stage as the curtains opened.

At first, when I thought the music was going to begin, the auditorium remained silent, and I got worried the music wasn't going to work at all. I stood onstage for almost a minute with no music, waiting, and the crowd started to cheer me on, thinking I was too nervous to do my dance, which wasn't true at all anymore—I was more than ready right when I stepped foot on the stage. The stage worker motioned for me to go backstage, and the curtains closed. Worried, I asked if the music was going to work, and they said they figured it out.

Pleased, I looked back at Jen, offering a small smile, which she returned. The curtains began to reopen, and thankfully, the music played. I started my dance, which began with sulking around, and finding a nearby bench to sit on. "Adrift" was performed to "Falling Slowly," which is a song from one of my favorite musicals called *Once*. The dance was sad; it told a story of a homeless girl looking for a family.

I truly danced my heart out onstage, earning very loud cheers and *Go Sarah Todd!*'s from the crowd. When I finished, I ran backstage and hugged Jen, both of us smiling widely. She had tears of joy streaming down her face as we walked out to the audience.

"When you were doing your long turn-combination, and everyone was going wild, I was silently praying that you wouldn't mess it up. And you didn't; everything was perfect!" Jen told me.

In the audience, I received many *congratulations'* and *good job*s. One of my friends' moms came up to me and gave me a big hug, also crying. She told me how great I did and how proud she was of me. I thanked her and went to see my parents, getting many more sweet compliments on the way. My mom and dad were very happy, and my mom was crying as well. Jen and I went to go sit with one of our favorite counselors, and, of course, she was also crying.

The reaction to my dance was unbelievable, and everyone who talked to me afterwards thought it was amazing. I was so happy that I was able to perform my solo, because it was the first solo I had ever performed onstage, and the first time I had performed onstage since getting Transverse Myelitis. It was a super special moment for me, and I know it was for the audience, too, as well as Jen. I kept wanting to go back on the stage and do it again since I had so much fun and felt so accomplished. It seemed that I had regained a lot of the confidence that I knew I had years before when I performed onstage all the time.

This was the first piece to the whole story—the beginning.

Performance.

Jennifer

"You have suffered enough, and warred with yourself..."

I held my breath, listening to one of my favorite songs without really hearing it.

"Raise your hopeful voice, you have a choice..."

I prayed hard that she wouldn't mess up as I watched a dance I'd seen a million times, without really watching it.

"Falling slowly, sing your melody..."

So far, so good. The dance was almost over, and she was doing incredible. Still, though, I didn't move a muscle from where I was sitting backstage.

Suddenly, I heard clapping and cheering. Loud clapping and cheering. She came running offstage, and I gave her a huge hug, both of us hardly believing she'd done it.

"And that was Sarah Todd's dance, 'Adrift!'"

Still more cheering as we walked from backstage into the audience.

"She choreographed it herself! That was amazing, Sarah Todd!"

I let out the breath I'd been holding since she'd first walked onstage. I realized that tears were running down my face as people came up to congratulate her.

It was hard to believe that I'd met Sarah Todd only a little more than two years before. I felt like I'd known her much longer; she was a little sister to me.

That dance was the first time in her life she'd performed a ballet solo. More importantly, it was the first time she'd really danced onstage since before she was paralyzed from the neck-down from Transverse Myelitis, when she was eight years old.

She was now twelve, only about two and a half months shy of thirteen.

Sarah Todd and I didn't live in the same part of the US—she lived in the south and I in the midwest—and we were four years apart in age. However, despite this, we had plenty in common.

For one thing, we shared a love and great passion for our hobbies. She enjoyed and was good at ballet dancing, while I loved to run track, cross country, and 5k races. This was probably why I loved watching ST's dances, the ones she choreographed on her own; I knew how much she loved it, and I was infinitely proud that she was able to do it.

Secondly, we both loved reading and writing. English was a subject we both enjoyed, and we loved writing random fictional stories.

The most important thing we shared, though, is the one that brought us together.

On April nineteenth, 2010, when Sarah Todd was eight years old, and on August sixteenth, 2011, when I was thirteen, we were struck by a rare condition called Transverse Myelitis, which paralyzed us both, amongst other sorts of problems. We'll be fighting it our whole lives, but we've also proven that we are more than capable of not letting it beat us.

"That dance was gorgeous," one lady said, tears glistening in her eyes as she squeezed Sarah Todd in a hug. I agreed; it was.

ST's performance was a huge step. Afterwards she continued to talk about how fun it was and how much she wanted to do it again.

At the same place and time only two years before, none of us would have thought that this would happen. Nobody would have believed that she would bravely step onstage in her sparkly gray dress, classic ballet tights, and pink ballet slippers and offer us a beautiful self-choreographed dance.

A lot can change in two years. It made me realize that although no big, noticeable changes had suddenly happened in that time, we were always changing and improving everyday nonetheless.

Determination

Part I:

2012

When they kept making gains with their passions—
Beating personal records in running;
Dancing improvements, in better fashion—
The girls knew even more wins were coming.
… Their first year of camp was a ton of fun!
New friends were met, who could often relate
To when they'd lost to life, and when they'd won;
A break to swim, to boat, to talk felt great.
Then in the girls' lives, new events went on:
High school began, a new chapter of life,
And doctors foreign as the amazon
Did tests; had ideas, plans that were rife.
And though the two met not a year before,
Their friendship continued to grow and soar.

Aspiration.

Sarah Todd

My DVD played soft music as I danced along to *Rapunzel*. I wasn't in this show like I should've been because of my TM that occurred a little over two years before. Despite this, I still memorized every single dance in the show.

I recognized many faces on the video, and it was cool to see my friends who were in shows with me at Atlanta Dance Theatre (ADT), be in the dance company and not be an extra. Being an extra in the shows was fun when I was little, but the parts were much smaller than the parts the girls had if they were a member of the dance company. Dancers usually had to be nine to audition for the company, and right before I got TM, I had reminded my mom to fill out the forms for the auditions. Even though I was only eight, my ballet teacher was letting me audition. I figured she probably wouldn't have let me if I wasn't going to make the company.

I couldn't help but to feel sad then because I should've been doing the classes, rehearsals, and shows with those girls. But, I was thankful I was able to dance again, at the very least. When I did the dances my friends were in, which I knew I would've been in if I hadn't gotten TM, I always thought about how much fun we had together in the shows through the years. I had known one of the girls in the dance I was doing since I was four, when I first started performing in *Babes in Toyland.*

That was always a very special show for me, because I was in it five times, and that show was something I knew I'd miss with all my heart; I had so many fond memories from all my performances in it. My first year in it, in 2005, I was four, and I got asked to be a toy duckling. This was very exciting for both me and my mom because only six girls total were picked to be the toy ducklings in the shows, for there were three in cast one and three in cast two. I was put in cast one, which meant I got to perform in the school show and two regular shows afterwards. After performing as a duckling, I knew I wanted to keep dancing in ADT's shows whenever I was given an opportunity. My love for performing grew because of the duckling part, resulting in me performing many years after that.

I continued in *Babes in Toyland* in 2006 up until 2009. In 2006, I was a Mother Goose child, as well as in 2007, just in a different costume, and I was playing a different game (all the Mother Goose children were playing outside, and in 2006 I pretended I was playing hopscotch; in 2007 I was chasing a butterfly with a net). I was so happy about my butterfly net part, because I got to do two leaps—or jetés—across the stage, which was great choreography for a seven year old because jetés take practice.

When I was in *Babes in Toyland* again in 2008, I was a snow fairy, and that part had its own perks, too. There were seven snow fairies in my group, and we held a snowflake in each hand while we danced and used them as props. What we all loved the most as snow fairies, though, was the fake snow—which was actually soap suds—falling onto the stage as we danced.

Lastly, in 2009, I was a gingerbread girl, which was a huge deal for me because the girls that usually received that part were nine or ten, and I was eight. Even though most of the audience's attention wasn't on the gingerbreads, I still loved the part because I was on the stage almost the whole second act. The costume for the gingerbread girls had to have been one of my most favorite costumes out of all the ones used in the show, which was a definite plus to the already-perfect part.

Babes in Toyland became a tradition because I'd been in it so many times, and every performance was special in its own way. I hadn't been old enough to be in any Spring performances my first few years at ADT, which saddened me, but that made performing in Babes in Toyland even more of a treat. However, when I was seven, I got to perform in *Swan Lake* in the spring. After *Swan Lake*, I chose to start auditioning for every Spring performance as well and was blessed with the opportunity to perform in *Cinderella*. *Cinderella* was the very last show I was in before getting TM, and also ended up being the last show I performed in on the Roswell Cultural Arts Center stage, less than a month before I got sick. I didn't know that after my last performance in *Cinderella* I wouldn't set foot on that particular stage ever again. My biggest dream was to have the leading role in an ADT show, just like my favorite dancer whom I looked up to and aspired to be like: Gia. She was Cinderella, and she smiled at me all throughout my magic fairy dance in the show.

When I was in the hospital, Gia had taken the time to visit me, and I was ecstatic. It had been an ordinary day at the hospital until I heard a knock on the door, and I mumbled, "I wonder who that is..." before I saw her. When I did, I pretty much screamed; I was very excited. She walked in with a smile on her face, and she answered the many questions I had always wanted to ask her about how she did stuff in shows. For example, in *Swan Lake* in 2009, she was Odette and I was a jester, and in one scene, she appeared in a birdcage that I was pretty sure didn't connect to a trap-door. So, I asked her about that scene that had left me clueless for over a year.

"In Swan Lake, how did you get in the cage?" I asked.

She laughed and then said, "I don't know," and shrugged her shoulders.

I never found out how she got in the cage, but the visit was fun nonetheless.

~~~~~

When Gia visited me, she revealed that ADT's next Spring performance was going to be *Alice in Wonderland*. The show sounded super fun to me, and I really wanted to audition for company after recovering enough to be in the show. I was a bit naïve to think that would happen, but I tried—in August of 2010, only about four months after I got TM, I went to ADT's open house for the start of the new dance year. My teacher gave me a big basket filled with ADT shorts, pants, shirts, a blanket, and many other small gifts. It was really sweet and made me feel welcomed back at my studio. I was very excited to get back to my old life as much as possible.

When I tried going back to my ballet and musical theatre classes at the studio when the school year started, which were the same two classes I had taken before, nothing was the same. Whenever the girls would go to the barre to do barre push-ups, I had to stand there and watch, there being no way I could do that activity. Although I didn't really notice, my balance was way off as well. Not that I could help it; I had just suffered a spinal cord injury not even four months before, and I probably looked very wobbly and noodle-ish. Of course when my dance teacher would look over at me and tell me not to try this move or that move—for example, the barre push-ups—I would earn weird glances from the other girls in my class, which wasn't that big of a deal, but it still bothered me. I did know for sure that word got around fast at my studio, though, so most of the girls probably had a little bit of an idea of what had happened—especially if they were in my ballet class when I started getting TM.

I ended up attending two of my ballet classes again after TM before I decided it was too much for me. This isn't something I would normally do, but it was very hard to do ballet without my arms and legs being normal. Yes, I could walk, but walking compared to ballet is extremely different—our bodies aren't naturally supposed to be able to do ballet moves, but we are naturally able to walk. My teacher was very sad that I quit, and I knew she would be, but I couldn't keep doing it. It didn't feel right, but I knew it would when the time came.

I kept attending my musical theatre class for awhile after, seeing as that didn't involve as much moving around. I stayed in that class for a few more weeks, but ended up discontinuing that one, too. It was too hard being there after just getting TM—I got frustrated that I couldn't keep up with my friends, and I got tired easily, which weren't good traits to have for an active class.

However, although I stopped taking classes at my studio, I still danced at home, where I continued to improve. I was slowly building back up to where I was before TM, and my goal after that was to become even better. I knew that if I kept practicing my dancing at home, I could be where I wanted to be and more.

It was only uphill from there.

Stubbornness.

Jennifer

I opened my eyes and saw that it was light out. I glanced at my clock, which glowed with the numbers "6:30."

I sat up in bed, rubbing my eyes as I awoke a little more. I got out of bed and dressed into a t-shirt and running shorts, then ran downstairs with a pair of socks. I was out the door and into the car by seven, tugging on my bright pink Lock Laces to secure my shoes as I waited for my dad to come into the car. He did shortly after, then drove me to the high school I would soon be attending.

When we arrived, I hopped out of the car and approached the field house doors, my dad walking right behind me. I took a deep breath and pulled them open.

I had run a little bit during the past few months, but not very much. Cross country camp every morning was going to help me improve. At least, I hoped so.

We found my soon-to-be coach and introduced ourselves. My mom had emailed him previously about my situation, the Transverse Myelitis that had paralyzed me less than a year before. My dad just handed him some paperwork and refreshed him on everything, then hugged me goodbye and left.

I stood on the steps awkwardly, hoping that someone I knew had decided to go to this camp, too.

Luckily, one of my friends walked in, and I breathed a sigh of relief.

When camp started, we did warm-ups, the lunges and leg swings that we would end up doing every day before we started. Coach then asked us to split into groups based on experience. Both my friend and I went into one of the lowest groups, for the relatively "inexperienced" runners. Or, in my case, the runners that *were* experienced, but recently had to relearn to walk.

A senior named Avery volunteered to lead our group.

As we slowly jogged for the amount of time we were supposed to for that day, Avery talked to us. She talked about her experiences in cross country and how she had been as a freshman.

It was really hot out, but I shrugged it off and listened to Avery as she spoke.

However, just then, we spotted a sprinkler that was watering the grass in a large field. Everyone kind of looked at it longingly.

"Follow me!" Avery said, turning and heading towards the sprinkler. She jumped through it, and the rest of us laughed as we followed suit.

The rest of the run flew by, and we ran a few hill sprints afterwards. When we got back to the school, we sat on the turf and performed stretches and exercises directed by Coach.

When I followed my dad to the car, I was ecstatic.

This is where I belong, I thought.

~~~~~

Four days a week, every week, I woke up bright and early for cross country camp. It was pretty much the highlight of my summer at this point.

One of those days, we were timed running a mile. Though the mile had never been my strongest race, I could run it in about seven minutes before TM. Today, of course, I was definitely not expecting to run it that fast; I just wanted to do my best.

Still, though, when I was done and found that I had finished in a little over ten minutes, I was a bit disappointed. I didn't want to be, but I really couldn't help it.

This would take more work than I'd thought.

Energy.

Sarah Todd

While checking my Facebook account one day in July, I decided to see if anyone was posting in the group I was in for teens and preteens with TM. Nobody had posted in awhile, so I decided to write a post asking who would be at the TM camp in Kentucky later that month.

Jen quickly replied saying she would be going and was excited for it as well. We had started talking the previous November, but had only just met in person that March. A few minutes later, our friend, Erica, commented saying she was going, too. I had met Erica that last October at a TM camp called Victory Junction, and she had brought Jen and me together the year before by recommending us as friends on Facebook. After I knew that those two were going, my mom told me that Annie from Baltimore would also be there. I was very excited to introduce Annie to Jen, and I knew we'd all have a fun time together.

~~~~~

After a long car ride with two brothers who wanted to watch weird movies, we arrived in Scottsville, KY. My parents checked us into the camp, and we collected our green nametags for the week since we were in the green lodge. I got more and more excited as we made our way back to the car; I couldn't believe I was actually going to see all of my very close friends who I hadn't seen in a long time—the week was definitely going to be a blast. After collecting our suitcases and bags from the trunk, we brought them into our "den," number eight. Our room had eight beds and nightstands, and a bathroom. Claiming my bed, which had one railing on the side of it and was closest to the bathroom, I set my pink ballerina bag on it, and eagerly approached the door, wanting to see who had shown up. Right when my mom opened the door for me, she pointed out a sign on the door right across from ours that read "CCK welcomes the Starzec Family!" I immediately gasped and got out my phone to send a text to Jen—I knew she would be extremely happy with our cabin placements.

There was a camp orientation in the gym that started at 5:30 that everyone had to attend, so I knew I would see her there. My family chose seats at the top of the bleachers, so I saved some for Jen and her family. However, I grew nervous when the orientation started and she wasn't there yet; I tried to pay attention to the camp director to keep my mind off Jen. Thankfully, my nerves died down soon after when I saw her walking in with her family, and we waved at each other. She and her family came and sat to the right of mine, then introduced themselves quietly while the camp director spoke.

The camp director led us in the CCK cheer, which I was very excited about. Everybody else seemed to do it sheepishly, while I did it very loudly with a bunch of enthusiasm. Doing the cheer reminded me that I was at camp and I was going to have so much fun, which is why I loved doing it.

After the director and counselors went over all the camp rules and regulations, Jen and I hung out in my room a bit before going to dinner in the dining hall. The counselors had us sit by cabin, which wasn't a problem for us since we were both in Green, and Jen and I had a great time chatting, laughing, and eating. After we ate, music started playing, signifying it was time to clean up and dance. I really wanted to do the dances like most children were, but Jen was having none of it, so I quickly gave up on trying to get her to dance with me: she would crack soon enough.

~~~~~

Throughout the few days at camp, Jen and I did many activities together. Some of them, though, we definitely did not want to partake in. One of those activities was the "Messy Games." This was where each cabin was a team, and there were different stations that contained extremely messy, gross activities, and everyone poured all the disgusting substances on one another. The kids who wanted to participate dressed in old clothes they didn't care about and wrapped their wheelchair wheels in plastic to keep them safe. Some parents even participated, which was really funny—especially because I was a kid and didn't want to do it. Our friends tried repeatedly to convince Jen and me to do it, but we really didn't want to. So, we decided to watch for a bit, which wasn't that entertaining. We were also worried that ice cream and other messy substances get on our clothes, so that made the Messy Games even more of an activity we didn't want to be involved in.

When we got bored, Jen and I went to the gym since no one was in there, and I decided to show Jen how to do some simple ballet moves. I started with the five basic ballet positions, showing Jen the way her feet should be in each one. Jen could do those while I demonstrated them, which made me happy, feeling accomplished. Wanting to see how far Jen could go with this, I decided to start teaching her harder moves. She could successfully do a decent arabesque, but doing jetés (leaps) was a different story. Watching her attempt the leaps was pure entertainment, and I guffawed when she stumbled and almost fell on the gym floor, like the good friend I was. I began to do them with her the more she fell, and she eventually got her front leg straight, which was progress.

Later, the Messy Games had finally ended, and it was time for everyone to clean themselves. CCK had a fire truck come and spray their hoses down on everyone, and after the fire truck left, everyone went to shower and go to bed. Jen and I stayed up later in the family room of our cabin, never wanting to sleep when we were with each other.

~~~~~

Jen and I went to the beauty shop the next day during the counselor activities, and we were greeted with the prominent smell of chemicals and soap.

"What do you want to try?" Jen asked me.

I looked at all the options, which were hair washing and dying, pedicures and manicures, and makeovers. "Let's look at the hair dye," I suggested. They didn't have many color options, and what I really wanted was pink, but I ended up choosing silver out of the choices I had. A counselor came and sprayed it in my hair, and I looked in the mirror, loving the way it made my hair look even blonder. Jen opted to get two French braids and no dye, and when her hair was done, she gave me a makeover.

That night, Jen and I stayed up late again, but we eventually fell into a peaceful repose, needing energy for the next day.

Joy.

Jennifer

Ding

I looked up from my summer reading book at the notification that popped up on my iPad.

"Sarah Todd Hammer tagged you in a post in the group *Transverse Myelitis Teens*"

I tapped on the notification banner, and my Facebook app opened up. It brought me to the group, and I scanned the top post.

"KY is next week... excited?! I know that Jen & I are!!"

I laughed after I read the post. I had only met Sarah Todd once in my life, just a few months before, but already I felt that we knew everything about each other.

She was 100% correct. I was definitely excited for TM camp in Kentucky the next week! It would be a long drive, but I could already tell that it was going to be more than worth it. I would get to see ST again, as well as meet some other kids with the condition, whom I'd recently been in contact with.

Another notification popped up, saying that one girl commented.

"I'm excited (-:"

She clearly wasn't alone.

~~~~~

"Are we there yet?" my little siblings whined, only half-joking. My mom sighed, and my dad answered as the GPS brought us to a long, winding road.

"About ten more minutes, guys."

Eight minutes or so later, my siblings started excitedly yelling as the Center For Courageous Kids sign came into view.

"We're almost there!"

I put my book into my bag and pulled out my phone. As expected, I had a couple texts from Sarah Todd.

"I'm in green cabin! I think you are too, in the room across from mine!" one read. I smiled, hoping that was true.

I opened up the next text, which was asking where we were. I already knew that we were cutting it close and probably going to be a little late, which made me pretty nervous... I really wanted to spend maximum amount of time hanging out with ST and other TM friends I knew I was bound to meet.

"We're here!" I texted back as my mom parked the car in front of the information building. My mom opened her door and walked around to the building to check in.

I jumped up and down in my seat in excitement when I saw her walking back to the car after what seemed like hours. She held a medium-sized white plastic bag in her hand.

"What cabin are we in?" I asked her, obvious enthusiasm in my voice.

"Green," she said as she tossed nametags to us in the back, which would be hung around our necks with green lanyards.

I slipped the "Jennifer" one over my head and handed the rest to my siblings as my mom drove to the cabin.

She parked the car in front of Green, where it would sit for the next five days.

~~~~~

After quickly transporting our things from the trunk of our car to our room, "den" number six (which happened to have a sign on the door that read, "CCK Welcomes the Starzec Family!".... It *was* across from the one that said "CCK Welcomes the Hammer Family!" after all, so I could see how Sarah Todd found out where I was going to be), we hurried over to the gym for camp orientation.

Orientation had started at 5:30. Right now it was 5:40, so we were a bit late.

One lady was talking as we slipped into the crowded gym. I scanned the bleachers, finally seeing Sarah Todd and her family at the way top. I waved and hurried up to sit by her.

Our families quietly introduced ourselves, and then we stopped talking and listened to the lady—who was actually the camp director—speak. She was now talking about the "camp cheer" we -would apparently be shouting often.

"Okay, now, let's try it! CCK, HOW DO YOU FEEL?" She yelled.

"WE FEEL SOOOO GOOD," the campers responded. "UH WE FEEL SO GOOD, UH."

Clap, clap, clap clap clap. Clap, clap, clap clap clap. Clap clap clap, clap clap clap.

"WHOO!" *Clap.* "UH!"

Sarah Todd did the cheer with as much enthusiasm as a ten-year-old could possibly have. I laughed, doing the cheer, but with a more normal amount of excitement.

"Let's try that one more time!" the camp director said, then recited the first part of the cheer. The campers followed suit with the next lines.

"WHOO! UH!" ST screamed beside me.

Empathy.

Sarah Todd

"You're recording?!" I squealed at Jen. Looking up at her in amusement, I began to do more frivolous things in front of the camera, which included dancing around like a maniac, and waving my arms about. Admittedly, being around my friends made me do highly bizarre things. A few minutes later, I even found myself walking around the room with a towel over my head, blocking my eyesight.

"What's this?" I asked Jen, putting my hands on something smooth and cold.

"A counter," she laughed. "Be careful. I don't want you getting hurt because I put a towel over your head."

"Yeah, don't worry," I told her, brushing her comment off and advancing forward some.

And... three steps later, I bumped my nose on the wall. Hard.

Jen laughed—of course, because that's what best friends do when the other gets hurt—before asking if I was okay.

"Yes," I mumbled, embarrassed, and clutched my sore nose.

~~~~~

Since we didn't want me getting hurt anymore, we decided to go hang out in the gym. We proclaimed the gym as ours—"ours," as in our hangout place. We even picked out a very special corner of the large gym—a corner where we could pursue all our shenanigans. Setting Jen's iPad up in our special corner, we made many more funny videos throughout our time at camp.

~~~~~

Of course, people usually eat three meals a day, so CCK had breakfast at 8:30, lunch at 12:00, and dinner at 6:00 in the dining hall, with snacks set up all day as well. After every meal, the camp counselors tried to get everybody to dance to some extremely loud music. I was always into doing this very much, while Jen wasn't. So, I had decided that I would make her dance because she hadn't cooperated the days before.

Getting up from the table we ate at, I pulled her arm over to where everyone was dancing. The music for the "Cha Cha Slide" blasted loudly through the speakers, and I danced along to the super fun song enthusiastically. Jen decided that she wanted to be a party pooper, so I tried pulling her over to dance with me. I thought it was ridiculous that she didn't want to; I quickly overcame that when the music turned off and we set off towards the oh-so-wonderful gym.

After a while, Jen and I got bored of the gym because more and more people kept coming in to play basketball, and we were too embarrassed to be our normal, crazy selves in front of them. So, we found Erica and Annie and took them back to the Green Cabin. In the front of the cabin was a huge family room that had cabinets (where games were kept), couches, and a fireplace. We set up Jen's iPad on the treasure chest in front of one of the couches, and I began making funny faces at the camera. The girls all laughed at me, and I cracked up at their reactions. Sometimes we played hide and seek, too, because that game never gets old no matter your age. If it was possible, Jen and I tried to hide together while whoever seeked—whether that be Erica or Annie—looked for us. There weren't very many hiding places in the cabins, which meant that we often had to reuse hiding places each time we played, so we couldn't play that for very long. We were so loud and probably annoying sometimes during the supposed "siesta" time that I was not very surprised when a few people came out of their rooms and asked us to quiet down a bit.

~~~~~

Even though I spent quite a lot of time at camp with all my friends, I still spent a lot of time with my family, too. I attempted to do archery with the help of my dad and went on a boat ride with my mom. Archery was extremely frustrating because I couldn't pull back to shoot the arrows, so my dad pulled back while I basically just held onto the bow, trying to make it feel like I was doing it. Going on a boat ride was more fun because the only thing that I needed a hand with—no pun intended—was getting into the boat.

Though TM camp was clearly loads of fun, there was one major downside: watching all of the children that have TM waist-down or belly-button down use their arms and hands. I knew it wasn't right to be jealous, but it was hard not to be, in that situation. I dreamt of being able to cut my own food, put my own shirt on, and scratch the top of my head normally, as well as many other everyday activities. Most of those kids could do those. But, they couldn't do a lot of things, too. Many couldn't put their own pants on by themselves—which is something I could do, albeit in a funky way; many couldn't get in the car by themselves which, again, I could do; and, most importantly, they couldn't walk. I knew what that felt like: not being able to get up out of my seat no matter how hard I tried, feeling like I was tied down with some sort of rope to a wheelchair.

Really, all that rope was, was reality. Reality of not being able to walk. Reality of not being able to move your hand or take a shower by yourself. Reality was, and is, the truth. When I find myself longing to be like the kids who got TM waist or belly-button down, I quickly remind myself to stop thinking that way, because my life would be so different if I couldn't walk. Of course, TM still stinks even though I can walk. But, even if I wanted it to be different, it wouldn't matter; I can't change reality, and reality can't change me any more than it already has.

One thing out of the many things TM taught me was that every time my chest rises and falls and I'm able to breathe, I should be thankful. Every time I take a step, I should be thankful. Every time I'm able to move *any* part of my body, I should be thankful, as should everyone else. Most people just don't realize this because each of these tasks goes unnoticed every time they are accomplished.

Oftentimes, the meaningless parts of our lives become the most important when they're lost.

Support.

Jennifer

"Wanna go to the gym?" Sarah Todd asked from behind me, jumping up and down in her usual post-dinner excitement.

I finished scraping the remnants of my meal into the trash and nodded.

"Let's go!"

"Yay!" ST screeched, flailing her arms around before literally doing pirouettes and jetés down the sidewalk connecting the two buildings.

"Calm down," I said, but I was laughing.

Finally, we reached the building that held the gym. I opened the door for Sarah Todd, and both of us ran in.

"Annie!" she yelled, running up to one of the other teenaged TMers whom I'd recently gotten to know. Sarah Todd had met her in Baltimore months before, and had introduced us on the first day of camp.

"Hey!" Annie said, giving Sarah Todd a quick hug. We sat in a circle—Sarah Todd, Annie, Annie's sister Kate, and I—and started talking.

"What's up?"Erica asked as she plopped down next to Annie in the circle.

"Nothing," ST replied. "Just talking."

"Well, they're setting up the fire in the dining hall right now. We can make s'mores soon," Erica informed us. Sarah Todd smiled mischievously.

"Oh boy," I groaned, fake-worried. "Sarah Todd and sugar do not mix!"

Everyone laughed and nodded in agreement. ST just jumped up and pulled on my arm.

"Come on!" she said.

"You want to go for s'mores *now*?" I asked. She shook her head.

"I'm going to teach you guys how to dance."

She proceeded to move her feet into the five ballet positions, gesturing at me to try it. I rolled my eyes, giggling as I clumsily copied her. Kate stood up and did the same.

"Good! Now let's jump!" she said, just hopping up and down in no specific manner. I shrugged at the other girls and followed suit.

"All right. Now that that's done... We go for s'mores."

Sarah Todd pointed towards the exit before skipping all the way to the sugar-filled dining hall.

~~~~~

I awoke the next morning to the sound of my siblings getting ready. I was exhausted after having spent almost all night hanging out and eating snacks with ST and our other friends.

"Jen, it's 8:20! You need to get ready for breakfast!" my mom shouted from where she was doing her makeup in the bathroom.

Sighing, I shoved my comfy quilt off and hopped out of my bed. I grabbed some random clothes from the dresser next to me and threw them on. After brushing my teeth and running a brush through my hair, I ran out of the room to where my mom was waiting to take me to the dining hall.

The sun was already hot when we got outside, even though it was only 8:30 in the morning. By the time we reached the satisfyingly air-conditioned dining hall, my face felt flushed and sweaty.

I scanned the room, looking for my friends. Sarah Todd's blonde ponytail suddenly bobbed into view as she followed her mom to a table. I sped-walked to the same table and sat in the empty seat next to her.

"Morning!" I said, already excited in anticipation of the day's events.

"Hey," she responded sluggishly. I knew that would change as soon as she was fed and awake.

Counselors passed bowls of food out to each of the five long tables. When they got to us, I examined the choices.

Eggs, bacon, potatoes, and fruit. I grabbed a little of each, except for the bacon, and passed them along to ST. She piled her plate with bacon and added a tiny bit of fruit.

"Got enough bacon there?" I joked. She giggled, sticking a piece in her mouth and biting down to create a satisfying crunch.

Music was turned on and garbage cans whisked out when the majority of the room was finished. After cleaning up, Sarah Todd danced crazily to the music. I stood on the side, watching her and shaking my head.

"Come on!" she prompted, waving at me. I crossed my arms in defiance and kept my ground. She rolled her eyes and continued dancing.

Finally, a Justin Bieber song came on, prompting the ten-year-old to cover her ears and fake wail. She dragged me out of the building, and we sat on the benches right outside and talked. Erica and Annie soon joined us. We talked for a long time, until our moms came out to bring us to the next activity.

"Let's see..." Mrs. Hammer said, scanning the activity schedule to see where we were supposed to go. "Green Cabin... there we go! Green and Yellow Cabins are scheduled for swimming."

The four of us cheered. Swimming was a mutual favorite for sure.

We ran to our respective cabins and rooms and quickly changed into our bathing suits. By the time my family and I got to the pool, Sarah Todd was already there and in the water, big goggles covering her eyes.

I grabbed my goggles and waded through the shallow end of the water to my friend, then held my breath as I plunged my head underwater. Sarah Todd did the same, and we waved at each other. I propelled myself to the bottom of the pool and felt the cool cement on my palms as I lifted myself into an underwater handstand, then held the position for approximately five seconds before my balance was swayed and my legs toppled into the water. I floated back to the surface, catching my breath.

"How did you do that?" Sarah Todd asked in amazement. I laughed.

"An underwater handstand isn't all that impressive."

"But can you help me do one?" Sarah Todd pleaded. I shrugged.

"I'll try!"

It was just recently that I had re-taught myself underwater handstands. Before I got TM, I had crazy good arm strength. I loved walking on my hands and doing handstands, cartwheels, and roundoffs, amongst other things. After my arms were paralyzed from TM, I could no longer do any of that. Needless to say, when my arms recovered enough to do a "handstand" with the assistance of a body of water, I was very happy.

I attempted to teach my friend, though it wasn't very easy. Most of the attempts resulted in fits of giggles as I got splashed. We eventually gave up on the idea and spent the rest of the time in the pool racing each other, talking, and playing catch with our other friends.

I woke up on the last day of camp feeling incredibly groggy. Erica and Annie had wanted to pull an all-nighter the night before. I wasn't sure if they succeeded or not; I had gone to my room to sleep at some point after midnight.

That day was sad. We had ice cream for breakfast, the talent show, and a mini carnival in the gym, but that was in-between packing and goodbyes. As we loaded our car with all our luggage at the end of it all, I looked back at the camp and all the good times it gave me. I was sad they were over, but couldn't wait for the new ones I had to come.

I gave my friends one last hug before we entered our respective cars and drove away.

Encouragement.

Sarah Todd

Sometimes, I felt a little bit down and discouraged about TM, but I knew it was only normal. Most of the time I'd have a huge smile on my face and would usually be happy. But, one day in August, I posted a Facebook status that said, "If TM hadn't happened, so many things would be different." Which, all in all, is most definitely true. If TM hadn't happened, I wouldn't know Jen or any of my other TM friends, and I would most likely be dancing with the company at ADT. I might even have had different friends at school, because the principal arranged my schedule with classes that were near each other, which of course meant that I likely would not have gotten classes with the same people.

It's funny how things work out sometimes. People's emotions become bottled up inside them and they need to get their feelings out. That's why I made that post on Facebook: to let people know how I was feeling and to see what they said. I didn't do it for attention, though it may have seemed that way to some of my friends. Instead, I posted that because I needed some cheering up; I wanted to see if my friends' and family members' comments could encourage me to think more positively about TM. Some of the comments ended up helping me think more positively, because they were telling me to smile and talking about how much I had recovered since being in the hospital for two months.

Although the comments lifted my spirits, I still no longer remembered what it felt like to lift my arms up high in the air; to feel my left hand in a fist. Just little things that I used to never pay attention to, because I had no reason to, would mean everything for me to do now. And, I was determined to do those things again.

~~~~~

At times, it seems like other people don't pay attention to my struggles, and it's only understandable; I don't exactly wish for others to know that my body doesn't work correctly. However, other times, people do notice, and I'm usually thankful for that. One day, in fourth grade, when I tried turning super heavy pages in my binder over, it took me a long time to get even some of the pages turned. I still had several pages remaining to turn when my arms and hand started getting tired, so I started to look towards my assistant to ask her to help me when one of my friends asked if I needed his help. I smiled at him, telling him yes, because I'd rather have one of my classmates help me than an adult for a change. He helped me turn the many pages in my binder so I was on the page I needed. I thanked him, and I was very happy that he stepped up and was a nice, helpful friend.

On the other hand, I don't really want people to help me *all* the time; I like to try doing things on my own from time to time. I do this because I might find a new way to do everyday activities such as opening applesauce, opening the refrigerator, brushing my hair, etc. For example, Jen once showed me how to open up a container of applesauce by stabbing the foil on top, which was one of many ways of adapting daily activities.

At my Welcome Home party after I was released from the hospital, I was sitting at the table with two of my friends and one of their moms, eating my food off my plate with my right hand. My friend's mom looked over at me and noticed how well I did with picking up the brownie and bringing it to my mouth. She commented, "Sarah Todd! That's amazing, you couldn't do that when we saw you in the hospital!" And, she was right.

Times when things such as that happen are wonderful, and I love it when people point out when I'm doing something that I previously couldn't. However, one thing that I really don't like is when I'm doing something a bit differently than most people would probably do it, and they just finish the task for me without asking if I need any help first. I understand that they're just trying to be helpful, but this irritates me greatly in some cases because I want to be independent and accomplish as much as I can on my own, even if I'm not doing it conventionally. As I said before, sometimes I appreciate the help, but most times, when I want help, I'll ask for it. If I don't, it is most likely because I'm attempting to accomplish a certain task in my own way.

When disabled people try to do more everyday activities on their own, it'll help them to be more independent as they live with the disability. For instance, I learned to put my shirt on by laying it out on my bed, then putting my left arm through the sleeve as much as I can get it to go through, then doing the same with my right arm. Next, I open the head hole wide enough so I can push my head through it, and then shimmy my shirt down because it may get bunched up at my chest sometimes. Learning how to do this made me increasingly independent as time went on, and it was nice for me to not need my mom's help with all types of dressing.

There are specific tools made to help disabled people do things, but those don't always work so well. When I went to the Medical Office Building (MOB) for therapy after I finished going to Day Rehab, my therapist had me try a tool to help me unbutton and button my shorts or pants since I couldn't do that with my hand. I tried for a long time to use the tool, but it never worked for me. So, I was left not able to unbutton or button my clothes still, leaving me to always wear clothes without buttons or ones loose enough to keep buttoned.

I progressively found new ways to do daily activities, and we had to get creative with some of them, like opening the fridge. Our fridge is hard enough for anyone to open because it's so heavy, so I wasn't *that* discouraged that I couldn't open it because it was to be expected. However, my dad brought home a wooden spatula from the store one day and showed me how to use it. I put it in-between the handle and the fridge then pushed out, causing the fridge to open. Hardly believing I could do it, I kept opening the fridge with the spatula over and over, very happy.

Since I needed more help in the kitchen other than with the fridge, we continued finding ways for me to be independent. All our sodas are kept in the fridge in the garage, which I could open without the spatula, and I could grab a soda out of that fridge, but I couldn't open the can. So, we bought an "easy opener," and I put the can's tab in the opener and pulled to open it. I couldn't hold the can with my left hand while I opened it, obviously, so I used the opener while sitting down and holding the can with my legs.

The tiny bit of freedom I gained made me smile, knowing more may come.

Diligence.

Jennifer

My feet pounded on the ground as quickly as I could manage without totally draining myself. I heard the shrill of Coach's whistle and breathed a sigh of relief, slowing down. I was already exhausted, but luckily only had a couple rounds left to go.

The whistle workout was used a lot in cross country camp. We ran slowly at first, then sped up for a little bit at the sound of the whistle. When it was blown again, we could slow back down. This repeated a few times. It was a tiring workout, but a good one. This, along with all the other workouts we had done throughout the summer, had improved me greatly. I was speeding up by the day.

A few days later, we had another mile time trial. I remembered my time from earlier in the summer—over ten minutes—and as a result, had some mixed feelings about this. I wanted to see how much I had improved, but was also a little scared of raising my expectations too much. Still, I couldn't deny that I was at least a little excited.

My friends and I arrived at the school at the normal time, bearing water bottles and granola bars, as usual. Some of the older kids brought spikes as well, but I didn't have mine yet. "Spikes" are special running shoes used primarily for racing in both cross country and track. They are thin running shoes with virtually no ankle support, and have a few holes on the bottom to screw tiny, metal spikes into. They are used to increase traction when running and make it harder to slip.

I tightened my ponytail as I nervously waited for my coach to arrive. Finally, he did, and we all pushed our way outside to start some lunges and leg swings. Shortly after, we momentarily parted ways for our warm-up jogs.

Before I knew it, the pre-run ritual was done and I was on the track, sipping from my water bottle. The kids with spikes put them on and laced them up, while the rest of us tightened the laces of our normal running shoes and got ready on the track.

I ran as fast as I possibly could, trying to give myself a good visual as to how much I had improved. I wanted to be able to compare the times and be both amazed and proud.

My lungs burned and my heart was practically beating out of my chest. I passed some teammates, and got passed by others. Finally, I had about 100 meters left of my final lap. I sprinted, gritting my teeth and slicing my arms through the air. Well, my left arm, anyway. I sliced my left arm through the air and made a sloppy attempt with my right.

I passed by my coach, and he yelled out my time. I barely heard it as I focused on slowing myself to a stop instead of toppling over or running into something. I stood in line behind the other finished teammates to get my time recorded by the assistant coach.

I ended up running that mile in around seven and a half minutes. It wasn't the best I had ever done, but it was a huge jump from the ten minutes only a few weeks earlier! I left the school with a big smile on my face, feeling like my running career was on the upswing.

~~~~~

As the summer came to an end, the school year neared. Usually this wasn't a huge thing for me, but this year frightened me. I was only days away from being a freshman in high school. High school! I already knew a lot of people from cross country camp, but the place still held a lot of mystery. I had no idea what kinds of things I would face; I would be treading into unknown waters.

In early August my mom and I went to the school to pick up my schedule and textbooks, and get my locker and combination. We were also going to get my gym uniform and such.

When we got to the school, we waited in line for a few minutes with a bunch of other students. We got to a lady sitting at a long white table, and my mom gave her all the necessary paperwork; in return she handed my schedule to us. I didn't open it quite yet, even though I was dying to.

We went to another lady at a similar table next. It was one of the school nurses. My mom explained my situation with Transverse Myelitis. She then asked if I could have two sets of textbooks, one to keep in my classrooms and one to keep at home, since I wouldn't be able to carry them around. The nurse was nothing but nice, and promptly gave us a note to hand to the bookstore lady.

The bookstore was our next stop. It was a little far from the area in the front where we previously were, and I started to get a little scared. The school already looked like a giant maze.

We waited in line again once we got to the bookstore. When we arrived there, we gave the lady my schedule and the note from the nurse. She nodded and gave me a huge stack of books. I looked at the covers as she piled them up on the table and counted. Twelve books total! I would've gotten six if not for the extra set: four big textbooks and two super thin ones. My mom paid for a gym uniform, lock, and heart rate monitor strap next, and then we set off to find my locker.

It was on the second floor. My locker, the locker I knew I would have to keep for four whole years, was on the end of the row, right next to an ancient-looking water fountain. I carefully turned the lock to the numbers of the combination I'd been given and popped it open. It wasn't incredibly difficult to open, luckily.

My mom helped me put one set of the books and my gym stuff into the locker, then swung it closed.

We ate at a Mexican restaurant afterwards. I opened my schedule there, looking at my classes, room numbers, and teachers. I didn't know any of the teachers yet, of course, but I was still interested.

Period 1: Advanced Algebra and Trigonometry Honors

Period 2: Freshman English Honors

Period 3: Freshman Girls PE

Period 4: Lunch

Period 5: Concert Choir

Period 6: Spanish II Honors

Period 7: Biology Honors

Period 8: World History Honors

Studying my schedule, it all felt more and more real. I was really, really nervous at this point, but I knew I could do it.

~~~~~

Freshman orientation came very shortly after. It was on a Monday; the older students were going to start that Wednesday.

I rode the bus for the first time in awhile. My friends sat by me, and before we knew it, we were at school.

All the freshmen gathered by the field house. There was a combination of familiar and fresh faces in the crowd. Everyone had the identical mixture of excitement and nervousness on their face.

This is more or less the group I will be with for the next four years, I thought.

Finally, we were ushered into the gym and sat on the bleachers. After a brief introduction, we watched upperclassmen play games with freshmen who volunteered. I found myself laughing more than I thought I would be.

We were told to find our name tags next, and joined a group led by two upperclassmen. We then spent time playing games, and having a tour of the school while dressed up in themed costumes. Advice floated everywhere throughout the day.

"Get involved!"

"Take your homework seriously."

"When I say get involved... I mean get involved!"

"Don't worry too much about a bad grade, just use it as a lesson to try harder next time."

It all seemed simple enough. By the time I was on the bus home, I could tell high school was going to be fun. I knew that there would be some difficult things, but overall it looked new and exciting.

I was no longer an eighth grader at that K-8 school I'd been going to for so long. I was now a freshman at this high school.

Strength.

Sarah Todd

One morning in September, I woke up and immediately noticed my scratchy, clogged throat. I tried to clear it, but I could hardly breathe. Because my lungs were already weak from TM, whenever I had a cold, it was awful—I couldn't cough up the phlegm in my lungs, and it made me feel like I was choking. This felt slightly worse than a cold, though, but I just assumed I had an awful one this time. Lying in bed all day wasn't something I particularly wanted to do, either, being that I was usually pretty active.

Getting through my sick days ended up being grim—I got bored fairly quickly when I couldn't dance. When I couldn't dance, I wanted to even more, and it became an endless cycle. However, since I was having extreme breathing difficulties I had no chance of being able to dance. Eventually, it got so bad that I had to stand in the bathroom with the shower on so that it'd create steam to help me breathe. Whenever I started getting that choking, breathless feeling back, I panicked and didn't know what to do; I definitely did not want to go to the hospital. But, when my throat began to hurt for the next few days and I developed a high fever, my mom knew she had to take me to see a doctor, which I definitely didn't want to do because I'd had my fair share of doctors already. It didn't help that, since getting TM, whenever I got sick, I automatically assumed something was seriously wrong with me.

I'm always worried doctors will want to order tests that will hurt or are unpleasant, so every time I see a doctor for something strange, I get scared. The doctor visit ended up being all right, though, which I knew deep down it would be, and we found out that I did have a bad cold in addition to an allergy to a plant called ragweed. I knew the whole ordeal wouldn't have been as much of a scare if I didn't have TM, but thankfully, everything was okay.

~~~~~

Later that month, my mom invited a few friends that we met at TM camp over for lunch. Erica, who was from Alabama, came with her mom and her brother, Justin. Another friend, Bridget, was from New Jersey, and her parents happened to be in town that weekend so they came as well. Even though Bridget wasn't able to come, I was still excited to see her parents and spend time with them. They came over first, then Erica's family arrived, and they spent a few hours with us eating lunch and chatting. We ended up talking a lot about TM, of course—sharing new info we'd learned since we last saw one another, and ranting about how ignorant some people are towards those with a disability.

Bridget's parents told us about a time when someone came up to them, pointed to Bridget, and said, "Excuse me, but what's *wrong* with her?" The question irritated them because the emphasis made it seem as if Bridget had done something wrong, when, really, the situation was quite the opposite.

Bridget's mom had replied vehemently, "Well, there's nothing wrong with her, but if you're wondering why she's in a wheelchair, then that's a different question."

Even though most people don't mind being asked about their disability, being careful with how questions are worded is a good idea so that they don't come across as ill-mannered. No one wants to be disabled—it's just one extra thing that we have to deal with. And, with the "one extra thing we have to deal with" (that being the disability), come many other extra things we have to deal with, even though we don't want to by any means.

For example, TM requires me to see loads of doctors every year, and because of that, I don't even mind going to simple appointments like the dentist, orthodontist, and pediatrician because I know every kid goes to them, and it's nice to go to normal appointments every once in a while.

One thing I know that for sure pesters those with a disability and their families is medical appointments, tests, etc. costing so much money. Because, not only do we have a disability we *don't want*, we have to spend tons of money on medical things we *don't want* for our disability. That just adds to our list of "extra things we have to deal with."

Willpower.

Jennifer

Freshman year started off exhausting, but I was having fun with the new high school experience nonetheless. I woke up at around 5:45 each morning, over an hour earlier than I had in middle school. I took the bus to school in the beginning, but as fall settled in and the weather grew a bit chillier, my friend graciously picked me up each morning. I was grateful for this, because although it was still pretty warm in the afternoons during the beginning of fall, it was frigid that early in the morning, which was hard to stand in for very long. Plus, who likes the bus?

After school each day, I excitedly attended Cross Country practices and meets. As the season went on and I raced more and more, my legs and lungs seemed to get completely better. My physical therapist told me that I still had weakness in my hips and core, but I knew that I was making gains anyway; the times I achieved at each meet proved it.

The first meet I ran was at a course that was full of hills. My friends and I walked along the path before the race started, and we grew increasingly apprehensive at the seemingly mountainous terrain. We named one of the biggest down-hills the "Raging Bull" of running—after the popular rollercoaster at Six Flags, Great America—and silently reminded ourselves that adding seconds to our final time by going slowly down it was worth it if it meant we avoided falling.

By the time we got back to where we had our stuff, the meet was just minutes away from beginning. We had accidentally walked the longer, 2-mile loop around the course instead of the 1-mile one, and as a result wasted a lot of time and nearly missed our race. We hurriedly changed into our uniforms and switched our regular running shoes for our spikes. I didn't yet have adaptive laces on my spikes, as they were brand new, so I let my mom tie a hurried bow onto each. My teammates and I ran to the starting line, and got there just in time. So much for thoroughly warming up beforehand.

"ON YOUR MARKS," the starting person yelled. All of the runners who were lined up jumped up and down and did some last-minute stretches.

"GET SET!"

Everyone froze in a starting position. Butterflies fluttered in my stomach in anticipation.

BOOM!

The sound of the gun went off at once, and my feet left the starting line immediately. The beginning stretch of the race was over fairly quickly, and the mob of runners thinned out as everyone found their natural pace.

I slowed up a hill, trying not to waste too much energy. I slowed down it as well, a tip from my coach: we naturally want to speed up at a decline, but that wastes unnecessary energy that will leave us exhausted later in the race.

All of a sudden, the laces came undone on one of my shoes. I immediately panicked, trying to keep my shoe on and also trying not to trip on the laces. I couldn't re-tie it myself, and no one could help me during the race. I felt helpless.

I heard my mom cheering for me as I turned around the corner. I looked at her with desperation in my eyes and pointed to my shoe. She returned my anguish, knowing that she couldn't help me. Nobody could. It was all up to me.

When I got back into the woods, I quickly knelt down and tucked my laces into the sides of the shoe. That was the best I could do to keep from tripping during the run. I stood back up, having successfully wasted only a second or two fixing my shoe, and finished the race.

My mom adapted my spikes that night. Though I'd managed to keep it on the whole time, I was delighted to know that I would not have that problem again in the future.

~~~~~

Our second meet was just days after the first, and I ended up doing pretty well in that one, as I ran the three miles in a little under 28 minutes. That was maybe a half a minute faster than the first meet. When it came time for our next race, I was hoping that the flat terrain and perfect weather predicted for that day would at least give me a minute or so off my time. If I could run it in under 27 minutes, I would be really happy.

When I and the rest of the sea of runners took off from the starting line, I remembered my coach's advice and tried not to go too fast in the beginning. The adrenaline and excitement of the beginning of a race makes you want to start off sprinting; however, that would only come as a disadvantage later on as fatigue sets in and lactic acid fills your joints.

I hardly heard my older teammates, coaches, and mom cheering as I ran. However, at one point I caught sight of another familiar face in the crowd: my physical therapist. She had come to cheer me on! I gained a boost of energy at that, knowing how much she had helped me recover. I couldn't help feeling like I owed it all to her.

All of a sudden, I felt like I was flying; I didn't feel any pain, fatigue, or anything. I felt as if I could run forever. A smile grew on my face, but that peaceful zone was broken when I passed by my grinning coach.

"If you're smiling, you're not running fast enough!" he shouted playfully. I just chuckled, and went around the bend to the last stretch of the race.

"Oh my gosh, go, Jen! You're doing AMAZING! Keep going!" I heard from the sides. It was Avery, the senior on the team whom I looked up to greatly; she was jumping up and down while loudly cheering for me. With that, I put my final burst of energy straight into my legs as I sprinted for the finish line. On the way, I happened to steal a glance at the clock showing my time.

"Oh my gosh," I muttered under my breath as I pushed myself over the line, then slowed to a stop. I grabbed my card with my place on it, but didn't pay much attention. I had run my race five minutes faster than the one before. That was completely unexpected.

A junior on the team gave me a huge hug when I got out of the chute, beaming. I was gasping for air, breathing harder than ever before in my life, but I was smiling. I felt amazing. I got more hugs and high fives from other older teammates, as well as from my mom and PT.

22:45. I had run three miles in exactly 22 minutes, 45 seconds.

"What was THAT, Starzec?!" Coach asked, grinning from ear to ear. I just returned the smile and shook my head.

This felt like a major breakthrough.

Dependability.

Sarah Todd

I had to take yet another trip to Baltimore. I definitely wasn't happy about having to take this trip at all, and Jen wasn't going to be there like the time before in March, which made the trip even less exciting. The Baltimore trip in March was by far the most exciting one, and I knew that it would be super hard to beat that trip.

Doing intense OT and PT every day with multiple doctors appointments in between wasn't exactly my cup of tea. Even though therapy wasn't something I preferred to do, my therapists did try their best to make it as fun as possible, and I appreciated that. My therapists always played games with me while I worked, and that made it less awful and boring.

My least favorite thing to do in OT (by far!) was ride the RT300 FES e-stim therapy bike—I already despised e-stim with a passion, but having e-stim on while my arms were attached to a therapy bike was even more horrendous. Part of why I went to Baltimore multiple times was because they had the bike, and the only place that had it in Georgia had a thirteen + age requirement. My parents really wanted me to have one to use at home, so they purchased one for me to use in my basement, but I absolutely didn't want to use it. Somehow, my mom ended up convincing me to ride the bike a few times a week while I watched TV. When I was in a particularly good mood while riding the bike once, mom and I named it Robert Timothy after RT300.

Over time, though, I stopped using the bike because I didn't feel like it was helping me at all. I knew if it did, the changes would be gradual, but the bike was too dreadful to use all the time. The way my hands had to be wrapped around the bars so they stayed made me feel like I was trapped and couldn't do anything for myself, which was a horrible feeling. Robert Timothy and I parted for months: until the next time I went to Baltimore.

~~~~~

Since Jen wasn't there that time, after all my appointments, I came back to the hotel for a snack and tried to find something good to watch on TV. The Homewood Suites had hardly any decent channels, so I usually ended up having to rule out watching TV and find something else to do to pass time. Sometimes I'd end up falling asleep and taking a nap because I'd had a long, tiring day at KKI, and I needed my rest. I tried not to do this a lot because a few times, when I did, I slept so late that my mom and I missed our dinner reservation if we had one, which was always a bummer. I felt bad about it every time it happened, but, hey, therapy at KKI was intense; of course I was wiped out! However, for that reason I tried ruling out naptime every once and a while, too.

Occasionally I would just lie down in my bed and play games on my phone or text. My phone that I had was an iPhone 3 that I used without data, meaning it was basically an iPod Touch. Because I had this phone, I couldn't use FaceTime since that application was only available on the iPhone 4 or newer. This always frustrated me to no end because I really wanted to FaceTime Jen when I became bored—even at home. Jen and I tried so many different video chatting apps like Qik Video and Skype, but since my old phone didn't have the front camera, those didn't work too well. On Qik Video, which was pretty much an older version of Snapchat, we ended up just messaging each other videos of us and our friends doing funny stuff sometimes. On Skype, on the other hand, neither of us could figure out how to work the video part of the app, and we only succeeded in making the chat part work, so we just deleted that app altogether.

One of those highly mundane days in Baltimore, I thought of a seemingly brilliant idea. My mom took her iPad with us to Baltimore for work purposes, and it had FaceTime on there. I asked her if she was using it, and she told me no. Beaming, I picked it up and flipped open the light pink cover. When I finished successfully typing in the correct passcode, I scrolled through the professedly endless pages of apps installed on the device. Once I found the light gray FaceTime icon, I opened up the app. I had never really used FaceTime before, so before I could call Jen, I had to figure out how it worked. Figuring out that I needed to select a contact, I swiped through them all until I spotted Jen's email address and phone number. I knew her email address was connected to her iPad, so I pressed on that one. Smiling, I waited for the words "FaceTime..." at the top under Jen's name to read, "Connecting..."

Just when I thought she wasn't going to pick up, the words changed to "Connecting..." and her face appeared on the iPad's large screen. I was so excited that it worked and that I wouldn't have to be bored for the time being, so I smiled and greeted her. Jen could sense my jumpiness and jitteriness, I could tell, so she laughed and said 'hey' back.

Trying to calm myself, I told her, "I'm so happy it worked! I can't believe I'm talking to you!"

The reason we were both ecstatic that we could FaceTime was because all the times before, we'd had to stay connected with each other just by normal phone calls and texting. The first time we called each other after meeting in person, we stayed on the phone for almost three hours, and I couldn't wait to talk to her for hours once again.

Jen smiled and nodded, saying she was excited it worked, too. She then asked me about my appointments and everything that was going on, and I told her all about my busy week so far. Then, we got onto the more interesting topics of conversation.

"Are you in the family room?" she questioned, leaning in closer so she could get a better look around the room.

"Yep! Oh, remember the bar we sat at?!" I asked her, gesturing to the two bar stools by the mini kitchen where we watched American Idol and ate Mexican food back in March. She nodded, and I moved the camera so she could see them.

"Bring back any amazing memories?" I joked since literally every piece of furniture or part of the suite in the Homewood Suites reminded us of some sort of silly memory from when we first met.

I continued showing her everything around our room so we could reminisce on our lovely Baltimore memories in the Homewood Suites that we loved oh-so-dearly. Talking to Jen for a couple hours on FaceTime that evening made it so I wasn't left with no activities to do at all, and it was for sure more fun than taking a nap and sleeping my life away.

Being able to talk for hours about literally anything that came to mind is something special I have with Jen that I don't have with any other friends because I see them all the time. Mine and Jen's relationship is more that of sisters, too, so we can tell each other anything we want and trust each other. No matter how many miles away Jen is, I know she'll always be just a text or call away if I need advice, someone to vent to, or someone to talk to, and I'm thankful to have a friendship as wonderful as ours.

Endurance.

Jennifer

Nobody was in a good mood the morning of this next meet, and for good reason: besides the fact that it was freezing and the temperature was expected to drop throughout the day, it was also the same day as our Homecoming dance.

Most people wanted to sleep in and have the whole day to get ready for the dance. However, we got a bit of a pep-talk from Coach and some upperclassmen beforehand, and tried our best to be excited for the race.

When we arrived at the course, I realized that the air was chillier than I had expected. I immediately remembered that I'd forgotten to bring warmer clothes to put underneath my uniform, which was starting to worry me a lot. Even with my sweatshirt on, I could feel the bite of the autumn air, warning us all of the harsh winter that was on its way.

Our tent got set up, and the underclassmen girls on the team got ready to start warming up, as the Freshman/Sophomore race was first. I kept my sweats on during the warm-up run, but still felt the cold seep its way into my skin, probably leaving goosebumps in its tracks.

When we finished, I followed the rest of the group to our stuff. We quickly changed into our uniforms and immediately threw our sweats back on over it, then put on our spikes. We then jogged to the starting line, where we did our remaining warm-up exercises.

The official came up, and everyone began to shed their sweats. I braced myself and waited an extra five seconds in the "warmth" before slowly taking them off. The wind, which was fierce, swept through me as soon as the extra layer was absent, making me shiver like crazy.

The gunshot rang through the air, and we were off, hoping to leave the chill at the start; if we were lucky, the exercise would cause heat to rush through our bodies. Maybe we'd even get hot!

Unfortunately, I never found that relief. It was too cold.

As I ran, the muscles in my bare arms and legs tightened up into a long-lasting, painful spasm. The strong, ferocious wind just made the chill worse, and as it blew around me, electric bursts of pain shot through my body. I automatically tensed, trying to preserve some heat. I already wanted to quit the race, and it had just started. But I wasn't a quitter; I knew I had to push through it.

My hands slowly began freezing up until I could not move them at all. They literally felt like blocks of ice, just dangling from my wrists. My legs started stiffening up as well, so I was basically running by just swinging them by my non-frozen hips.

Finally, the race was over, and I was able to breathe a huge sigh of relief. My mom brought me my sweats, some gloves, and a blanket, and tears streamed down my face when she did. I immediately felt very embarrassed when some fellow teammates noticed and gave me hugs. I hated the attention, and really just wanted to curl up under the covers in my bed at home.

However, I couldn't; it was against the rules to leave meets early without getting permission in advance. Since both of our tents had apparently broken during my race due to the wind, I lay out in the field next to my backpack curled inside of a sleeping bag for the remainder of the meet.

I couldn't help but hate TM on that day. It had caused me unnecessary pain and discomfort during a race that I could have done well in. However, I wouldn't consider it amongst the worst days of my life; the sun eventually came out and the wind died down, and the outdoor Homecoming pictures that took place that evening were painless.

~~~~~

The cross country season my freshman year was one of the best summers/falls of my life! However, it eventually had to come to an end.

I learned that there was a banquet at the end of every cross country season. During these banquets, we ate food, hung out with the teammates we'd grown so close to during the last few months, watched a slideshow, and received awards.

When I got to my school's cafeteria on the day of the 2012 cross country banquet, I immediately scanned the room for my friends. I couldn't find them at first, which made me feel very anxious for a second, as I hated how awkward I probably looked, standing there while looking around feverishly.

Finally, I caught a glimpse of my friend Fabi, and noticed she was sitting with a few other friends. A huge wave of relief immediately washed over me.

Even though I'd been in high school for many months by now, I was still in ninth grade; I wanted to blend in as much as possible and avoid further perpetuating the "awkward freshman" stereotype.

"Hey, Jen!" My friends greeted me as I sat at their table. I smiled and waved 'hi' back.

"Go ahead and grab some pizza!" Coach announced to the room, and everyone immediately rushed over to where the food was. I giggled at how excited everyone looked, but their enthusiasm wasn't surprising; they were runners, after all, and there's not much a runner loves more than food.

"Why are you eating your pizza that way?" one of my friends asked another friend, giggling as she did so. I looked over to see what she was talking about, and sure enough, she had folded her pizza in half lengthwise and was eating it that way.

"It's a pizza taco!" our friend said, and we all laughed. Soon, everyone was trying to come up with different ways to eat pizza.

In the end, we found that there are five different ways of eating pizza: the "normal" way, the "pizza taco" way, the "pizza sandwich" way, the "crust first" way, and the "pizza croissant" way.

The rest of the night went by very quickly. Coach put on the slideshow, which contained tons of pictures from the entire season. We laughed at all of the photos that captured my teammates goofing off in practice and at meets, and teared up at the sweet ones that showed the friendships that had developed that year, and how our team had turned into a family.

By the end of the slideshow, I felt incredibly sad that such an amazing season was over. However, I was grateful for all of the memories cross country had given me so far, and I was excited to see what the next season would bring.

Next, we received awards. Each freshman was given a piece of paper that said "Freshman Numerals" and his/her name on it. We also got little patches that said "16" (for our graduating year: 2016) that go on letterman jackets. I didn't plan on ever buying a letterman jacket, but I knew I'd find a place to keep the patches as soon as I got home.

The older athletes got different patches and pieces of paper, and then special plaques—such as awards for most team spirit and most-improved that season—were given to certain people. At the end, our coach said something special about each senior, and gave the "Four-Year Award" to each 12th-grader who had been in cross country for all four years of high school.

I smiled then, thinking about how desperately I wanted a four-year award. I definitely planned on continuing cross country the next three years, and the thought of getting that award my senior year excited me. I couldn't wait until I was an upperclassman and could be a role model to the future freshmen and sophomores, just like this year's seniors had been amazing leaders for me.

And, just like that, the banquet was over. My first year of high school cross country was finished.

I found my mom, and we began walking out of the cafeteria. However, Avery —the senior I'd looked up to the most that year—stopped me.

"Here, Jen. I'll miss you! Keep up the good work. I can't wait to see how far you get next year and beyond," she said, handing me a thick, white envelope with my name on it. She gave me a hug and walked away.

In the envelope was a folded-up piece of pink construction paper. I unfolded it and began reading the note:

"Dear Jennifer,

It has been great getting to know you this season! I know we haven't really had any intimate talks, but I've watched you really grow as a runner this season. You are for real, no lie, no joke, gonna be awesome by senior year. Stick with it! Winter training, summer training, everything. You have so much talent! That [22:45-meet] was awesome. My freshman year I ran [the races in] like 30 minutes then broke my leg, and last week, I ran at state. You are already so much better than I was, so think about it. I really hope you stick with XC for four years. I wish you the best of luck for the next three seasons, and hopefully I can come back next year and see you tear it up!

Love,

[Avery]"

Decision.

Sarah Todd

Ever since I got TM, my parents have ensured that I receive the best care possible and that I see the greatest doctors. Of course, this is a good thing since I don't want to see bad doctors; however, we have to travel for many of my appointments, and I greatly dislike it.

Evidently, all the doctors I need to see aren't in Georgia, so my parents took me to Greenville, South Carolina to go to the Greenville Shriners yet again for more appointments with the group from Philadelphia Shriners. We tried to make sure that we always could see this group in Greenville instead of in Philadelphia because we could drive the short three hours to Greenville in lieu of flying to Philadelphia, which was doubtlessly a plus.

Despite the Greenville trips being much less of a hassle than the Philadelphia trips, I never wanted to go on either of them or to any doctor for that matter. Of course, this was understandable, but I still needed to see all the important doctors, which I was not happy about.

When I arrived at the Shriners hospital in Greenville with my parents, we parked our car in the garage and took the elevator up to the lobby. The lobby was rainforest-themed, and it had waterfalls and huge animals everywhere, which placated me because the amazing decorations made it seem less like a hospital.

After checking in at the front desk and having my wonderful patient bracelets put on, we went to the X-ray waiting room. Since there were a lot of people waiting their turn, all of the seats were taken, so we ended up standing in the hall for about an hour. I had gotten used to waiting excessively long times just for an appointment or test that would take no more than fifteen minutes, so I wasn't surprised. When a nurse came out and finally called my name, she led us back to a room for an X-ray of my spine and left wrist. The doctors wanted the X-ray of my spine to monitor my scoliosis and the one of my wrist to monitor my growth plates. They monitored my growth plates to see how much growing I had left to do in order to determine how severe my scoliosis may get. Typically, scoliosis goes haywire during a growth spurt, and I hadn't reached mine yet.

The X-ray itself didn't take long at all, as I knew it wouldn't, and afterwards, we moved on upstairs to the clinic for my appointments. We ended up waiting well over an hour upstairs, and I quickly became bored and restless. For once, I was glad when it was my turn for my two appointments.

First, I saw the scoliosis doctor. He took a look at my back to see where the curves were, and then he showed us my X-rays. After looking at them with my parents, since I didn't really understand much of what he was telling us, he declared that there was only a two percent chance the curve would worsen. This was great news because the scoliosis wouldn't just heal itself; it would either stay the same or worsen. Therefore, hearing him say that certainly felt like a weight was lifted off mine and my parents' shoulders, and we were relieved there wasn't a big chance the curve would regress. He informed us there wasn't any bracing that would work to prevent my scoliosis from worsening because it's in my c-spine, which is highly unusual. Braces annoyed me to no end anyway, though, so I was relieved that I wouldn't have to wear an awful soft collar.

~~~~~

Tendon and nerve transfers often help TM patients regain motion back in certain limbs, so my parents wanted to see if this was an option for me. A good, working tendon or nerve could be surgically transferred to a muscle that's having trouble working, and over time, I could possibly regain motion back in that area. The whole idea of surgery terrified me, seeing as I'd only had one in the hospital before, and I wasn't up for the appointment. I disliked whenever we discussed a serious topic during doctor appointments that I didn't feel like talking about and felt like I wanted to cry because those types of discussions overwhelmed me.

This seemed to happen even more than usual with this doctor because the whole point of seeing him was to discuss any available tendon transfers, which wasn't something I was eager to have done. He brought up an idea to make my right thumb work better for grasping and doing a thumbs-up, and those motions weren't very important to me—I wanted something for my left hand. My parents thought it was a pretty decent idea, yet I didn't want to pursue this idea because I already had a little bit of grasp and thumbs-up in my right thumb. If his idea was for my left thumb, I would've considered it more because I could've gained function on that side. However, since I already had function on the right, gaining a little bit more didn't seem like a big deal to me at all; hence why I was so insistent on not doing this particular tendon transfer.

Eventually, while we were talking about the transfer during my appointment, my thoughts got all over the place; I thought about having to do surgery, having to get bloodwork done before surgery (if I did one), and how my hands should just work without a surgery. One thing led to another, and I began to cry. I always felt embarrassed when I'd cry during doctor appointments—or in front of anyone, really —so I tried to stop, but I couldn't help myself. Mom asked me why I was crying, of course, and I told her that I didn't want to do the transfer. I'm sure she probably wondered how I made my decision so fast, but I was adamant on not doing any sort of tendon transfer. I knew I would've had to do tons of intensive therapy to get my body used to using the tendon in a different way, and since I couldn't have the surgery at home because the doctors weren't in Atlanta, I would've had to have it in Philadelphia and stay there for a couple weeks for therapy. That would've been a major bummer to be away from home and in the hospital again.

The biggest reason why I absolutely did not want to have the tendon transfer, though, was because I would've had to wear the cast on my right hand for three months, meaning I wouldn't have had a hand for that amount of time. Since I wouldn't have had any hands to use for three months, I wouldn't have been able to attend school either, which meant that this had to be done in the summer. Doing this in the summer would mean I couldn't swim, too, which would've made my summer extremely boring.

The doctors and nurses were trying to convince me to go with their idea, and my parents were as well; they kept telling me that three months wasn't a long time to go through without my hand if it'll work better in the long run. Although I knew three months wasn't a long time compared to my whole life, I didn't want to—and still wouldn't want to—need help with *every* single thing I wanted to do for that long. Doing this surgery basically meant that I'd have no freedom for three months, and that was a lot to take in. I decided right on the spot that I didn't want to do it.

Most people probably would think that I was stupid for not taking up a doctor's offer to want to help me gain some function; however, if it was they losing independence for months and doing intensive therapy for weeks, I think they'd understand. If the surgery proposed was an idea for my left hand, I might've been hankering to pursue it because it could've helped me a lot, and I most likely wouldn't have lost any function from the limb where they would've taken the tendon. Unfortunately, that wasn't an option.

One of the things I'm glad that my parents allow me to have since I can do most thinking for myself, is an opinion on things like this. Because I didn't want this surgery, my parents didn't make me do it, although they still let it be an option for the future as the doctor said it didn't have to happen right away. Obviously, if I was younger than nine, I most likely wouldn't have been able to make my own decision on this, but I think that since I could understand most of what was being discussed at age eleven, it was nice being able to express my feelings about the idea. My parents clearly want what's best for me, so, even though they might not have agreed with my decision, it was what I wanted, and I was happy with my choice. I still wished he had an idea for my left hand, but there wasn't any luck that time.

Stamina.

Jennifer

I had been looking forward to the Hot Chocolate race for months. It would be my first 5k race since the summer—before Cross Country—and I was excited to see how well I would do. I was racing with a bunch of friends as well, so I knew that no matter how well I ran, it was going to be fun.

We had to wake up annoyingly early to get to the city in time for the race. We were carpooling so that only a few cars had to make the trip, so a bunch of friends piled into my family's giant car before sunrise. The ride wasn't terribly long; going early meant that we were able to escape at least some of the annoying Chicago traffic. That hour or so was spent resting a bit, since we'd woken up so early, as well as drinking plenty of water and Gatorade. We ate some protein bars, bananas, and peanut butter sandwiches as well, but not too much. Running had a lot to do with preparation, and all of us wanted to do it well.

When we got there, we laced our shoes and stuck our numbered bibs onto our shirts with safety pins. We then quickly went to the bathroom before heading over to where the race was.

The air was chilly, but I made sure to be prepared for that. I wore two long-sleeved shirts, which were both meant for running, so they were made from a warm but breathable material. I also wore long running leggings, gloves, and a hat. I hoped that it would be enough to keep me warm enough during the race, but not so warm that I overheated.

My friend and I stood in the huge crowd in the second group. The groups were released to start in order, and you were grouped based on how fast you were. The fastest people went first, and the slowest last.

We jumped up and down the whole time, partially because we were excited, and partly because we were a bit cold. I stretched my legs, doing a few different lunges I had gotten used to doing every day in Cross Country, so that they stayed loose and warm. The race was introduced, music started to play, and the first group, group A, was off. Only a few short minutes later, it was our turn to cross the starting line. My friend and I excitedly began running, immediately matching the pace of our group. We sped up a bit and passed a few people, finding a clear gap in the crowds that could be our own space.

The cold air did make my limbs stiff at first, but not quite as much as it would have without the warm clothes. The sun eventually came out completely, too, which warmed the air up a bit, and with it, my body as well.

The race went like any other, besides the huge crowds of people and the promise of chocolate afterwards. I enjoyed the experience immensely; I hadn't run in the city in a while, and I had a great time doing so. Downtown Chicago can be gorgeous, even if you've been there millions of times.

Besides the view, the experience was also amazing in other ways. As aforementioned, the race was a big one. I had never done one so popular before, and being able to run alongside so many people was pretty fun. Plus, there was music at some spots, which created a more uplifting, energetic mood.

As the race went on, I started to get really hot. I tore off my left glove and stuck it into my tiny pocket before rolling my sleeves up, but there really wasn't much I could do; I didn't have a pouch or bag or anything like that. Luckily, the air was still chilly enough that most of my body felt fine. However, I could feel that my feet were beginning to overheat.

My feet always seemed to overheat first. Sometimes it was random, and I'd have to randomly rip my shoes and socks off while in the car even in the dead of winter or wrap them in a cold washcloth in the middle of the night. Other times, of course, it was because I was exercising or it was hot outside.

This particular time, though, I was fortunate that the race was almost over. We heard cheering and louder music and knew that the finish line was quickly approaching. My friend bolted without hesitation, and I quickly followed. Her sprint was much better than mine, so she got there first, but I wasn't too far behind.

I crossed the line, breathing heavily and feeling slightly nauseous, both usual sensations at the completion of a race. The finish line held even more excitement, and I was able to ignore the aching in my body because of it.

Long white tables were set out on either side of me, and each was covered in little squares of chocolate. I eagerly took a handful and stuck it in my pocket. Other tables held fruit, water, and gatorade. I grabbed a bottle of water and gulped it down, quickly diminishing my thirst.

My friend and I sat by one of the fences separating the racers from the people watching and waited for the rest of our party. I took my hat, shoes, gloves, and outer shirt off, but it was only a few minutes before my body heat went down and the air felt cold once again. I layered everything back on except the hat, which had gotten annoying. My mom, who hadn't participated in this particular race, came behind the fence and handed me a sweatshirt, which I graciously accepted. I gave her the hat in return, which she threw in her bag.

Slowly, the rest of our group began to appear. Once everyone had finished, we got a picture together at the end and left the finishing area to consume some more chocolate.

After a bunch of laughs, full stomachs, and faces covered in chocolate fondue, we were all very glad we had the chance to experience that race.

Part II:

2013

Their strength continued to slowly improve,
And running and dancing got easier.
Each girl had something she wanted to prove—
After hardship, they knew they'd respire.
Jen became increasingly speedier;
She had a race soon and had to prepare.
But, as it grew colder and breezier,
Her cold muscles and nerves began to flare.
Frustrating dance moves were so much to bear,
And, though Sarah Todd always did her best,
Sometimes, it was difficult not to care.
Still, she loved ballet and danced with much zest.
Many didn't get their struggles or fight—
They tried to make those stereotypes right.

Poem by Sarah Todd Hammer

Effort.

Sarah Todd

Finding easy hobbies while having TM could be a bit hard, but I wanted to try new things as best as I could. When I was little, I baked with my mom a lot, so I decided I might benefit from trying it again. Baking hadn't always been a major hobby of mine, but I enjoyed doing it from time to time. Since I was little before I got TM, I needed assistance with most tasks during baking. One of my jobs whenever my mom baked a cake was cracking the eggs and blending everything with the mixer.

However, since getting TM, I couldn't do those things very easily, if at all. In order to crack eggs, I needed two working hands, and to mix the batter, I needed an arm that wouldn't tire out within 30 seconds of mixing.

Although, my mom found a recipe for some Valentine's Day pretzels that have melted chocolate kisses on them with Valentine M&Ms on top, which seemed like something I could help her make. She got the idea from Pinterest, of course, and showed me the picture of them. I thought they looked quite cute, so I was excited about making them with her.

I didn't realize that baking could be considered therapy, but that was a good thing, because I had fun while doing it. First, Mom started me out by having me read the directions to her on the website with the recipe. Successfully doing that, I walked back from my mom's desk to the kitchen counter where she laid out all the crucial ingredients: a bag of square-shaped pretzels, a bag of peppermint flavored chocolate kisses, and a bag of multi-colored M&Ms.

We needed to preheat the oven to 350 degrees so that we could melt the kisses into the pretzels. Our oven is pretty high up in our kitchen, so I couldn't reach it, but I was determined to. Since I could only lift my arm up to my ear, I pulled it back and swung it up high in the air, trying to grab the handle on the top oven. The first time I missed the handle, so I tried once more, achieving my goal. Once my hand grasped the handle, I carefully inched my fingers up to the buttons. I pressed all the correct ones and hit start, smiling because I could add something to my list of things I didn't need help with. Unclasping my hand from the handle, I let my arm fall back down by my side.

After I preheated the oven, Mom began opening all the kisses while she instructed me to place the mini square pretzels in a six by five array. Taking the pretzels out of the bag was exercise in itself because of how small they were, and I got good practice with picking up small objects. When I finished completing that, I grabbed chocolate kisses and placed one in the center of each pretzel. I was grateful that my mom unwrapped all the kisses for me because that would've taken me forever to do, and that job could've gotten quite tedious.

When the oven beeped, signaling it was finished heating, Mom took the tray of pretzels and kisses and put it in the oven for around two minutes because we only wanted the chocolate to melt slightly. When the oven beeped signaling the two minutes were up, Mom opened it and pulled the tray out, setting it back on the counter carefully. Then, she opened the bag of multi-colored M&Ms so I could place one on top of each pretzel. After finishing the whole project, my arms and hands had for sure had a great workout, and I was proud of myself for helping. It certainly felt great to be able to help with baking, which I hadn't had the opportunity to do in a long time.

~~~~~

It had been a few months since I'd seen my TM friend Erica, and I was beginning to miss her a lot. I heard about tons of things she had been doing recently, one of those activities being wheelchair basketball. Her mom told us she had a game in Marietta, GA, which was only about 45 minutes away from my house, and we thought about trying to go see her play. We thought it would be really fun, so my mom asked Erica's mom to give us all the details so my mom, dad, and I could attend. I was super excited to see her and her family, and I couldn't wait until the day she had her game.

My parents and I went together to see Erica play a few days later in Marietta. It was interesting to watch wheelchair basketball rather than regular basketball because the players played pretty roughly at some points during the game. The wheelchairs they used had wheels that stuck out a bit more so it was easier to push them and move faster during the game, which was part of what made the sport more rough. Some of the kids crashed into each other's wheels, and sometimes I was afraid that someone's wheelchair was going to tip over. Thankfully, that didn't happen, and nobody got hurt during this particular game.

After Erica's game, we talked about all that went on during it, and I told her I thought it was good that she found a sport that she learned to love, and she was good at it. Of course, wheelchair basketball wasn't something I would've qualified for or even wanted to do because I'd never been sporty. I reminded myself that I was lucky I wasn't sitting in a wheelchair at that moment and that I could go home and dance if I wanted to.

Erica and I had talked about how we thought we'd rather our TM to affect us, since it was bound to, anyway. After seeing TM kids walk with crutches at CCK for a few days, it had me thinking.

"I'd rather have TM like you, Erica," I'd said to her while sitting in a chair in the family room of our cabin. When I said this, I hadn't gone over what having TM like Erica would mean for me. I knew I missed using my arms so much that I thought I was willing to give up my legs for their use, but I wasn't. Every person with TM, I'm sure, sometimes wishes it had affected them differently. But, if we were able to change how it affected us, we'd definitely want to revert back to how TM originally affected us after the first day. I reminded myself it was wrong to be jealous, too; I surely didn't want to be wheelchair bound—I was thinking about using arm crutches to walk.

"Really? I'd rather be like you," she told me, acting surprised that I thought wanted to have TM the way she did. It surprised me that someone would rather not have use of their arms and hands than her legs, but then again, she was surprised that I thought I'd rather have use of my arms and hands with weak legs. I think we both knew that there wasn't much point in wishing to have TM a totally different way because that would never happen; however, we both liked thinking up scenarios in our minds sometimes. I knew the only reason we thought we'd want to trade with each other was because we're opposites—she has the use of her arms and hands, and I don't; I have the full use of my legs, and she doesn't.

"Sarah Todd, you wouldn't be able to dance," Mom reminded me, and that made me go silent for a minute, thinking everything over. I guess the thought of being able to do things I couldn't do (using my arms) made me want to give up the use of my legs since I was accustomed to using them. But, I figured that after a few hours of sitting in a wheelchair wanting to dance and not being able to, I would switch back to how I am in a flash. And, maybe Erica thought the same way, too.

"That's true," I finally replied, not being able to think of a repartee.

"The grass is always greener on the other side," Mom concluded.

Fortitude.

Jennifer

"Mom, s-s-slow d-d-down," I pleaded, teeth chattering. We were in the parking lot of a strip mall, walking from the car to DSW so I could exchange a pair of boots I'd gotten for Christmas, which didn't quite fit. My mom was almost at the entrance to the store, while I lagged behind. It was January, which meant it was *cold.* It seemed as if every muscle in my body was spasming and tightening up so much, I was incredibly stiff and could barely move. My knees were also collapsing a bit, making the walk even harder. Besides all of that, my fingers and toes were numb and tingly, even though I was dressed very warmly—thick socks, snow gloves, and all—and we had yet to be outside for more than a couple minutes.

I remembered the winter of 2011, right after onset, and how different it was. Back then, I could barely feel the cold, for whatever reason. In fact, I was walking to school one day in late-fall and was wearing a t-shirt, unaware of how cold it was until I saw that the people passing by were wearing winter coats.

Oh, how I wished my body's reaction to the cold had stayed that way, instead of flaring up 20 different symptoms as soon as the outside air hit my skin.

I dragged my legs across the parking lot, wanting nothing more than to just be inside of the heated shoe store. My mom waited for me on the sidewalk in front of the entrance and looked at me with an expression I couldn't quite read.

"People who don't see you every day have a hard time understanding how on some days—good days—you can run three miles, but can barely walk across the parking lot on other days," she said quietly.

"I know," I responded.

I did often wish that more people understood the invisible side of things. Even the people that seemed to understand, didn't really. However, I suppose it *is* kind of a strange concept to wrap your head around.

~~~~~

When January approached, the weather had gotten colder and colder, so more and more time passed since I'd last run. Because of this, as winter break came to a close I became excited for the indoor track season to start.

The winter was very hard on my body in general, but the vast majority of its effects were when I was outside. I just hoped that doing the running and workouts indoors would be okay.

On the day that indoor track began, my friends and I eagerly awaited the ending of our final class period. When it finally happened, we changed quickly before heading to the English hallway, which was where we knew the track team was meeting to start practice.

The track coach came in and introduced himself before splitting our group into sprinters, throwers, and distance for warm-ups. I was 100% a distance girl, but they often practiced outside, where it was way too cold for my body and messed-up nerves. So, I had decided to practice indoors with the sprinters and run the distance races at meets. It annoyed me to have to practice with starting block when I wasn't even going to need them and be practicing speed more than endurance, but it was what I had to do until the weather warmed up. Anyway, it was likely still going to improve and benefit me in many ways.

Our warm-up routine in track was quite a bit different than it was in cross country. In XC, we usually just did lunges and leg swings before each practice. In track, on the other hand, we had a longer routine with a bigger variety of different exercises. It wasn't what I'd grown used to, but I couldn't deny that it woke my legs up.

Our coach explained our workout once our warm-ups were done. In the past, I had done workouts similar to the one he was explaining, but not that exact one. I was excited; workouts were definitely exhausting, but some of them could be really fun.

"First, you guys will run really quickly down the English hallway," he said. "Your speed should be just a little bit slower than a sprint. At the end of the hallway, you'll slow down to a normal running pace and finish a lap around the second floor at that speed. When you get back to the English hallway, you'll speed up, and repeat the whole thing a few more times."

I ran with my friends, and for the most part, we kept each other's pace. I knew that pain was inevitable, especially considering we were inside our school; running on hard linoleum is hard on anyone's shins and knees. However, I was having a good time, and it felt nice to run after my winter hiatus.

Breathing hard and muscles burning, we finished the workout. We had survived our first day of track.

My friends and I walked outside to wait for our ride. I was bundled in my winter coat because I always froze and stiffened up at the first touch of cold air, but a couple of my other friends were hot enough from practice and went out in their t-shirts, carrying their coats in their arms.

"I can't wait for the rest of the track season! It's going to be so much fun!" one friend exclaimed. I thought so, too.

~~~~~

I did not feel well at all.

That was my first thought when I woke up that Monday morning. Mondays were never pleasant, of course. After all, with all the stress going on in high school, the weekend was a much-needed breath of fresh air; Monday always seemed to not only take that breath right back, but add a few extra pounds to my shoulders as well.

This Monday, though, was a bit different. I'd had chronic pain in general since August 16th, 2011 due to TM, but the achiness in my legs and upper body was way worse this morning. The weather had been pretty constant, so I knew it probably wasn't temperature change; I brushed it off as a random flare and got out of bed to start getting ready for school.

First period was math, and I grew nervous that my teacher would shove something at us that required a lot of effort, like a quiz or an extensive worksheet. Luckily, that didn't seem to be the case.

"Take your notes out," she said as she turned on the projector. I breathed a sigh of relief. I didn't have to do much of anything today; when my math teacher projected the notes for the rest of the class to copy down, she usually gave a copy to me so I didn't have to try to keep up with all of that writing.

I kept my gaze at the front of the classroom, trying to pay attention to the equations we were being taught to solve. They were probably important, but I couldn't focus. It wasn't even 8:00 in the morning and the day already felt long.

Finally, loud music filled the building, telling us that class was over. I rushed out of my math classroom and headed down the hall to my next one.

Second period. English.

"Good morning! Hopefully you all read that chapter over the weekend, because, as you probably remember, we have a reading quiz today. You have the whole class period to complete it," my English teacher said right after the bell rang. The class groaned as she handed the quizzes out. A wave of dread washed over me.

It was only a couple of pages long and didn't look difficult at all. But the ache in my arms grew to a sharper pain, especially in my left, which was the one I wrote with. I looked at the questions, but couldn't focus at all, and even holding the pencil hurt my hand.

The fifty minutes crawled by slowly. I tried as best I could, writing a few shaky sentences to answer some of the short response questions. Finally, the period ended. I sat in my chair as the classroom emptied, staring at my quiz. It was incomplete, and the answers I had completed were barely even legible. I was not going to get a good grade on this. And, more importantly, there was no way I was making it through the rest of the day.

"Jen? Are you okay?" My teacher asked as she walked up to my desk. That was the worst question I could be asked at that moment, because those words broke the dam holding me together, and I burst into tears, saying something only semi-coherent about my arm pain and lack of focus.

Luckily, she caught the overall point of what I was trying to say and brought me straight to the nurse, assuring me the whole walk there that I could re-do the quiz another time.

~~~~~

Strep throat. That was what was causing me immense pain that day: a simple bacterial infection that is easily treated with antibiotics.

I was glad it was that simple. But, at the same time, I was frustrated that it had seemed so complicated. Why didn't I have a sore throat or fever? Or even nausea? I had no classic symptoms, nothing indicating that I was sick. All I had was pain. The only thing telling me something was wrong was an increase in Transverse Myelitis symptoms. Now, because of TM, even having a mild, everyday illness was complicated.

I ended up having to stay home from school the rest of the week. When I got back, I faced a *lot* of make-up work, which was a little stressful. I wasn't feeling miserable anymore though, at least; the fact that just a few days of antibiotics cured this setback was a good thing I couldn't ignore.

Patience.

Sarah Todd

Even though I still thought I didn't look all that great while I danced, I thought that my skills and technique were much better than they were before I got TM, which was my goal. Dancing with a spinal cord injury is a challenge like no other, but I aspired to prove to myself that I could still be a phenomenal dancer even with a SCI—maybe even better than before TM.

I, of course, continued with ballet, but also tried different types of dance I'd never attempted before such as lyrical and contemporary, growing to love even more styles of dance—not as much as ballet, though! My grandma, Katie, asked me countless times if I had considered going back to take dance classes at ADT again since my passion for dance hadn't strayed, and my answer was always no. Katie really wanted me to get back into learning new moves in classes and boosting up my technique, but I explained to her that I could do dances older girls did and that I felt was fine on my own.

And, it was true. Since getting TM, my dancing improved each day, and I got great exercise when I did it. I focused a lot on my legs because I could do all the

120

moves with them; however, I usually let my arms do their own thing and didn't pay much attention to them at all. Jen suggested that I try to incorporate my arms into my dances more, and at first, I thought that would be impossible because in most of the moves, my arms would need to be above my head or higher up than I could lift them. But, she insisted that I should at least try, and Katie did, too. So, the next time I danced, I tried doing first position with my arms, which was where they were level with my belly button in a circle. My arms looked a bit crooked, especially my left one, but my right hand looked exactly how it should. It was funny: even though my right hand wasn't perfectly normal, my fingers still went into the correct ballet formation I'd learned at age three. Dance moves were like riding a bike for me.

I tried a few other positions with my arms, yet I wasn't happy with how some of them looked as much as I was with some others. In my arabesque, my arms had to be pretty close to my head, which I couldn't fully accomplish; instead, I put my arms in the correct position, but I placed them closer to my waist. When I did arabesques in the air, I sort of swung my arms up (much like I did when trying to reach the buttons on the oven) because a ballet move in motion is performed much quicker than a stationary one. Experimenting with different ways to dance with my arms was sort of frustrating, but I reminded myself that I would look better while I danced if I practiced them.

~~~~~

I had been dancing a lot to ADT's 2011 recital DVD, and I chose a few dances to learn and perfect. The theme for the recital was classical dance, which had several types of ballet. When I start learning a dance from one of my DVDs, I pick one girl in the dance based off where she's placed on the stage; if the girls did different moves at different times, I pick a girl who did my favorite ones. That way, while I learn a certain dance, I can follow one girl and not feel as if I have to watch all the dancers.

Once I memorized the dance, I worked to perfect it and get all the moves the way I wanted them to look; whether that be graceful, fast, or jumpy. Sometimes I changed some of the moves I didn't like or didn't think flowed well to make the dance easier for me to do; however, I didn't do this very often because if I started doing the moves I wasn't great at, I'd get better at doing them.

The dance I chose to work on started off with five dancers around twelve years old doing basic ballet in pointe shoes while dancing with a cane. After the five girls finished their dance, around ten older girls came on dancing in pointe shoes wearing hats that they took off and used as props. When both routines were over, all 15 dancers did a number all together.

Katie was over at my house with me while my family went out somewhere, and whenever Katie was over at my house for any reason, she asked if I had any new dances to show her. I decided to show her the dance I had been perfecting because she was always eager to see a new routine. Since I had the dance memorized, I faced away from the TV, so I could perform the dance facing Katie.

As the music began, each dancer turned around to face the audience, so I did exactly what they did.

I used some of the new arm movements I taught myself in my dance to see if she'd notice and for additional practice. Of course, after my dance, she told me how well I did, and she made a comment on me using my arms more than usual. I was glad she noticed because that meant the time I spent improving my arms had paid off.

She noticed that the dancers used a cane as a prop and asked, "Have you ever thought about using a yardstick as a prop because they're using a cane?"

"No, I don't think I'd be able to make that work," I explained, not really liking the idea of trying something I didn't think I'd succeed in. But, I knew if I never tried anything, I wouldn't be able to accomplish anything new.

"Let's see you try it! Go find the yardstick," Katie protested, trying to motivate me.

"Okay," I gave in and scampered off down the hall to get our yardstick. As I walked back to the family room, I imagined myself dancing with the yardstick as a prop, and I couldn't see it ending the way I wanted it to.

Katie watched from the couch as I started the dance over again, but with my new addition. The dance went pretty well from the beginning until I started having to move the yardstick over my head, hold it with two hands, and switch it from hand-to-hand. I began to grow extremely frustrated with everything: myself, TM, and the stupid yardstick. Abruptly, I stopped dancing and dropped the yardstick on the floor.

"I can't do it," I announced, going over and sitting on the couch next to Katie. The video was still playing, and I let it, although I didn't know why. It seemed as if the able-bodied dancers were mocking me. "I should be perfectly capable of dancing with a stupid stick," I grumbled.

As I said this, Katie still sat on the couch, and I got up to retrieve the yardstick off the floor. When I looked up after bending down to pick it up, my eyes met Katie's, and I noticed she was silently crying.

"Are you okay?" I queried, instantly worried that something had happened to her.

She looked up at me and said, "I'm just really upset you can't do it."

Of course, I was, too, but there was no way we would've been able to make dancing with the yardstick the way we both wanted possible.

~~~~

I learned to not be reminded of TM every time I had to complete a task differently or when I couldn't do something. I didn't think about TM every moment, and I knew that was a good thing. Of course, there were still times where it brought me down—everyone with TM has those, I believe—but, I'd learned to live with the way things are. There was no point in dwelling on it, because, what was there to dwell on? Even if I found out why I got TM, I would still be living with it every moment of every day. And, there was nothing we could do to change that.

While Mom and I were taking our dog, Buddy, on a walk through the neighborhood, the topic of TM came up, which happened occasionally. Mom still wanted to know why I got TM, but not knowing didn't really bother me. The thought never occurred to me on its own, but when Mom brought it up, I didn't delve into it all that much. This was simply because I didn't think knowing why I got TM mattered because even if we knew why I got it, I'd still have TM, and there was no changing that fact. TM happened for a reason, I believed. I just didn't know that reason yet.

During our walk, when we reached the park in our neighborhood that had the playground, basketball court, tennis courts, field, pavilion, and trail to walk on, Mom asked me, "Do you remember that day when you came home from school in second grade saying a ball hit your neck at recess?"

I thought really hard to see if I remembered that happening. "I guess so," I shrugged. "What about it?"

Buddy had stopped to take a break, so we stood where the park's parking lot was on the sidewalk, waiting for him as we talked.

Mom pulled on Buddy's leash, trying to get him to walk again. "Do you think that maybe, *that* caused TM? The ball could've hit your neck hard, and maybe something in your spinal cord freaked out."

I didn't really think that was feasible, so I told her that.

I turned away to start walking again, but she stopped me. Turning around, I said, "I don't want to talk about it. It doesn't even matter to me, anyways."

I hated that we had to have these conversations, but mostly, I hated how discouraged she looked; I also hated how all I could say was, "I don't know."

Guidance.

Jennifer

Anyone who has been to the Chicago area during springtime knows how incredibly unpredictable the weather can be. One day it can be below freezing and blizzarding, while the next it is sunny and warm enough to go outside without a coat on. Sometimes, multiple extremes can even happen in the same day.

Unfortunately, because of Transverse Myelitis, extreme weather often confuses and irritates my body, causing my nerves to go haywire and give me the loveliest gift: a flare in symptoms. Rainstorms make me extra fatigued and achy; too much heat causes my feet to feel as if someone dipped them into open flames. Humidity makes me drowsy and makes moving my arms and legs more of an effort, while freezing temperatures make my fingers and toes stiff and numb, amongst many other things. When these weather conditions appear suddenly and drastically different than the day before, these symptoms are even worse.

Chicago springs are usually awful, sparking a war inside my body. The only thing that makes them better than our winters is the occasional days of perfect warmth and the knowledge that summer is approaching.

The spring of 2013 was no different. By the time April rolled around, I was completely exhausted from the long winter and ready to skip right to June. That is, until my mom informed me that we were taking a week-long trip to Texas to visit some Transverse Myelitis specialists at UT-Southwestern. It was going to just be me, my mom, and her best friend Cathy. I hated going to doctors and hospitals and getting tests done, but the notion of warm weather excited me enough to look past these negatives.

The day I was leaving for the Texas trip finally came after much anticipation. It was an especially gloomy day; the sky was as dark as if it was still nighttime due to an abundance of black clouds. It was raining, and I covered my head with my hands in a feeble attempt to stay dry as I ran from the car to the entrance of my school.

Still, despite looking like I'd just taken a shower with my clothes on, I was happy. I only had to suffer through a few classes before my mom picked me up to go to the airport.

~~~~~

"Hi, Jennifer!" A man said as he came into the room. We had been in Texas for about two days now, and we'd barely gotten any sunlight due to what was, in my opinion, an excessive amount of appointments. Though the weather was a huge relief after coming from gross Illinois, our Texas trip meant way more appointments and tests than I'd previously anticipated. Today, I knew I was going to be hanging out in the hospital all day; the day before had been a few hours of that stuff, too, including an annoying VEP Vision Test early in the morning. Still, the few times we'd gotten out in the sun made it feel worth it… At least a little bit.

"Hi," I responded shyly, shaking Dr. Greenberg's hand. I vaguely recognized him from TM camp less than a year before but had never really talked to him.

A team of doctors was in the room by now, and they immediately started spouting information, asking questions, and evaluating me. None of this was new to me, of course; I was used to all of doctors' evaluations, such as testing my strength and reflexes. I was used to answering all the usual questions about my onset of TM, pain levels, biggest difficulties each day, and more. I zoned out when I responded to them, my answers all but scripted at this point.

However, I was a little surprised when one of the doctors told me to stand up and lean forward after I mentioned my chronic back pain. He pulled the back of my shirt up a little bit and examined my back before telling us that I had thoracic scoliosis. I would need to follow up with an orthopedist to get X-rays regularly and monitor it, even though the scoliosis was pretty mild at this point, and the chance that it would get too much worse was slim. It was likely due to how badly TM had weakened my core; because of the weakness, I had a hard time sitting or standing straight.

I was glad I had an answer for the back pain, at least, even though there wasn't much of anything we could do to fix it at this point.

~~~~~

"We want to repeat some of the neuropsychological testing you had done in Baltimore last year."

I groaned when one of the doctors said that a little bit later. The year before, I had gone to Johns Hopkins and the Kennedy Krieger Institute in Baltimore for a few different tests and appointments. One of the things I did there was a grueling two-day-long neuropsychological test, which had concluded that though I was very smart, I had cognitive slowing from TM, for some unknown reason.

I still struggled with finishing tests at school even with extra time, so I didn't think I needed to repeat the neuropsych tests; they probably wouldn't show much of a difference. I looked at my mom and mentally pleaded with her to not make me do that again.

"It won't be nearly as long as the other one, Jen," my mom said. I sighed, still not incredibly excited about it, but I followed the doctor into the other room, anyway.

This neuropsych test was almost exactly as I remembered the Baltimore one to be, just a bit condensed. After what felt like 12 hours of puzzles and memory games —but was probably less than two—I was able to leave that tiny room and re-join my mom in the other one.

I didn't get much of a break, though, before a team of doctors came filing into the exam room again.

They said they wanted to talk about pain management, which wasn't a huge surprise to me. When I was first in the hospital from TM—way back in August 2011—the doctors had talked to us about starting a medicine called Neurontin. However, my mom and I had decided not to, because I hated meds, and we figured my neuropathy would eventually get better.

But now, almost two years post-TM, it was definitely not better. If anything, it was worse than before.

The doctors discussed all of our options with us. They mentioned so many different types of pain meds, like Lyrica and Nortriptyline and Cymbalta. In the end, though I really wanted to be open to trying new medicines, I was too leery of the potential side-effects. However, I filed the information away in my mind for future reference in case my pain got less bearable.

The next thing they wanted to do was talk about a tendon transfer. The spot in-between my thumb and index finger on my right hand had almost no muscle, so my thumb was incredibly floppy. That thumb worked a little bit, but really only moved up and down; that little bit of movement didn't help me that much, because my thumb didn't have the movement it needed to be stabilized and grip things. Because of this, I wore a little blue brace on that hand, which stabilized my thumb enough that I could hold some things. The brace also protected that spot with very little muscle, because it was incredibly sensitive.

The tendon transfer they were suggesting would likely make it so I wouldn't

need to wear that brace anymore, and my thumb would gain some more movement,

which might make that hand a bit more of use. However, I decided that I really

didn't want a tendon transfer; surgery was very scary to me, even though it wouldn't

be a huge one, and I didn't want to go through a whole surgery and a bunch of extra

therapy just to get a tiny bit more use in that hand. I'd already adapted to the

movement I had and had figured out ways to do most daily tasks, so I was almost

completely independent despite the partial paralysis.

Besides, the brace worked just fine, and I didn't mind wearing it every day. I

knew that tendon transfer surgery was a great invention, and it helped so, so many

people; it just wasn't right for me at the time.

After that, our appointments were finally over. However, we couldn't leave the

hospital quite yet. The doctors asked us if we wanted some of my (anonymous) test

results to be used in their TM research. We agreed to that and went downstairs to

get blood drawn so they could use those results in their studies. Though I didn't

particularly like blood draws, I was definitely used to them and hoped my results

would help with their research.

~~~~~

The Texas trip ended up giving us a lot of new insight. The many tests and

examinations I did over those few days showed that I had scoliosis, cognitive slowing, mild hydronephrosis, and some other things. Even though it was a long week, I couldn't deny that they'd helped us quite a bit.

And, of course, the weather wasn't a bad addition.

134

Inspiration.

Sarah Todd

My parents always wanted to explore every possible opportunity they can for
medical treatment, which was why I was constantly dragged to different places all
around the country such as Greenville, Philadelphia, and Baltimore many times.
One place we had not been to was Minneapolis, and my mom wanted to take me
there to go see some doctors at the Mayo Clinic to discuss more possible tendon
transfers. We had basically stopped hoping there'd be an available nerve transfer
because we'd been told that those were only best to do before reaching the one year
anniversary of TM.

The day before we were going to leave, I sat by our pool with my dad, telling
him I really didn't want to go to Minneapolis, and he told me, "Think about this: in
two days, it'll be over, and you'll be back at home." That made me feel a lot better:
knowing I'd be home soon. So, I sat there by my pool, wishing I could stay there
instead of leaving.

The flight to Minnesota wasn't that bad, but there was no flight to Rochester,
which was where we needed to be for my appointments. So, we flew to

Minneapolis and took a shuttle for an hour and a half to Rochester after the flight, which made traveling way more stressful and tiring.

Once we checked in, Mom told me one of our other TM friends who had been to Mayo before told her about an underground subway that they really liked to go to. I thought this was a bit weird at first because when I thought about an underground subway, I immediately thought of the subways in New York. I'd never been there before, but I'd seen them in movies, and they didn't look nice at all to me. But, it turned out that the underground subway was a way for people to get to the Mayo buildings without having to go outside since Minnesota could get extremely cold in the winter. It was nice being there in July so we didn't have to worry about freezing to death; it was even warmer there than it was in Atlanta, which was weird.

The subway turned out to be a really cool place to go because there were tons of fun shops and restaurants down there and it connected to our hotel. So, we went down there to explore the shops and restaurants when we arrived, then we went to our room to relax. Our hotel was really nice, and I was super happy that we were finally there so I could lie down to rest. Traveling really takes a toll on people with spinal cord injuries.

After we gained more energy from resting a bit, we wanted to get dinner somewhere, so we asked someone at the front desk which restaurants were good. We decided to go to a pizza place down the street after the worker at the desk said it was good, and I was excited because I loved pizza. The place ended up serving really tasty pizza, and I enjoyed it very much. During dinner I talked Mom's ears off about One Direction and all their latest gossip, but she didn't understand most of it. It was still fun gushing about all of them to her, even if she didn't totally understand the hype.

~~~~~

The next morning, Mom and I walked through the subway to get to Mayo. I was immensely surprised at how nice the inside looked because it surely didn't look like a hospital at all—it was satisfying to walk in and not immediately smell the typical hospital stench, and everything there was clean and overall beautiful. Most of the employees looked happy to be there, and everyone we talked to was helpful and personable. The friendly environment made me less nervous for my upcoming appointment.

We found where we needed to go for my appointment, took the elevator there, and went to the waiting room. After waiting for a while, me playing "Draw Something" on my iPhone to occupy myself, my name was called, and we went back to see all the different doctors at once. I tried to mentally prepare myself for the stressful, chaotic appointment I was to endure—I greatly hoped I wouldn't feel like crying during this one.

When we got situated in our room, the doctors and my mom started talking about tendon transfers, and I sort of tuned it out because I got bored quickly. But, I started paying attention more when the doctors thought of the same idea for my thumb that the doctors had in Greenville. The topic, of course, made me upset again because I definitely didn't want to do that surgery.

Thankfully, we moved on from that idea pretty quickly when they thought of another one: they could take a tendon and move it to my right shoulder so it'd be more useful. This suggestion didn't sit well in my brain because the doctors said since my shoulder is so tiny and hardly has any bulk, it would look like I had a big ball of muscle sitting on my shoulder. I didn't want my looks to be involved in the transfer in any way, so I almost immediately ruled out another idea once again. I had to will myself not to cry again, because thinking about possibly having that surgery done upset me—I didn't want to do it.

After our appointment, the doctors recommended we go see another doctor we weren't scheduled to see, which I wasn't happy about. We had to go to a different part of Mayo to see him, and we ended up waiting over an hour. Waiting wasn't as bad as it could've been, though, because Jen and I were texting about publishing *5k, Ballet, and a Spinal Cord Injury* since we had finished writing it a few weeks prior. I was getting jittery talking with her about it, but that ended when my name was called; I was relieved to be done waiting, but I didn't desire to listen to or discuss anything medical. While I sat in our room and listened, Mom talked with this doctor more in depth about the possible shoulder surgery. When that was done, I was extremely grateful I could go back to the hotel and rest after a tremendously long day. Remembering we had scheduled a shuttle to take us back to Minneapolis so we could get up early and fly back home the next morning, I groaned. Sitting on a shuttle for an hour and a half was the last thing I wanted to do after those appointments.

~~~~~

On the shuttle to Minneapolis, I texted my dad and some friends to pass the time—I still couldn't wait to plop down on my bed in our new hotel. I was relieved when it was our turn to get off the shuttle, even though it was the last stop the driver made. We had to take a train to get to our hotel, though, so we weren't done traveling quite yet as I'd hoped. I noticed a lot of girls getting on the train, but I didn't think anything of it before we got on—on the train, there were girls wearing 1D shirts and face paint.

Looking over at my mom, I whispered, "I think those girls are going to a 1D concert."

She seemed clueless and said, "Really? Look up and see if they're here."

I eagerly pulled my phone out, searching "1D tour schedule" and scrolled through all the dates. After a bit of searching, I finally came across the correct date: **July 18, 2013: Minneapolis, MN**.

"Mom! They're here! In Minneapolis!" I grumbled, annoyed my favorite band was in Minneapolis the same day we happened to be and I wasn't getting to see them. *While thousands of girls are watching their favorite band perform live, I'll be sitting in my hotel room*, I thought. That was what I'd thought I wanted to do. Not anymore.

"You're kidding!" Mom sounded surprised. "Maybe we can go and see if there're any leftover tickets."

I wasn't completely sure that was possible, but I figured she wouldn't have suggested it if it wasn't. Hearing my mom say this made me go from glum to overjoyed, and I couldn't wait to be off the train. I had never been to a concert before, and I thought it'd be amazingly cool if 1D got to be my first.

When the train finally made it to our stop, we rushed off and found our hotel. After checking in, we went up to our room and quickly charged our almost dead phones while changing into more decent clothes. The whole time, I had so much adrenaline pumping through my veins because of how eager I was to find the arena, but at the same time, I was anxious because I didn't know if we'd find tickets or not. We checked the hotel room's clock and realized we had to leave then if we wanted to have enough time to get there without being late. After getting off the elevator, we walked outside the hotel and pretty much just followed all the other girls to the arena.

Once we reached the outside of the arena, I saw a guy holding up tickets saying they were for sale, so I told Mom, "Look! Let's buy those, Mom!"

She quickly shook her head, "No. Those might be fake."

She grabbed my hand and led me towards the doors that had big signs saying "SOLD OUT," which made my heart fall.

"Let's just go inside."

When we got inside, there was a huge crowd of people trying to get in the correct lines to officially enter. I was super confused as to why we were still there after seeing the signs, and I knew we weren't allowed in without tickets.

"Mom, the sign says sold out!" I informed her, still immensely confused.

Pulling me through the colossal crowd, Mom said, "Let's just follow these people." Giving in, I let her guide me through everyone. Once we were in a line, I grew worried.

"Mom! We don't have tickets," I cried. "What're we gonna do?"

Right as I said this, though, Mom smirked and pulled two tickets out of her purse as I squealed. I hugged her while she laughed, and I started crying because of how shocked and surprised I was. I never thought I'd get to go to a One Direction concert in my life! But, the surprise got even better when the worker told Mom where our seats were, and I instantly screeched, "You got floor tickets?!" as she nodded.

We found our seats, which were very good, but I mentally scolded myself for not packing a 1D shirt. I was a huge fan at a 1D concert, and I was wearing a cookie shirt, which made me very embarrassed. Although, all that embarrassment faded away when I was watching my favorite band perform live, and two of them waved to me a few times. I couldn't believe Mom had cooked up such a huge surprise without me finding out, and after the concert, I was definitely glad we'd gone to Minnesota.

After the amazing concert was sadly over and Mom and I were in our hotel room, I thanked her a million times and scrolled through all the pictures and videos we took. Mom explained to me the only date the Mayo doctors could see me was July 18th, and that just happened to be the day 1D was in town. This wasn't a coincidence—everything truly does happen for a reason.

It certainly was the best moment of my life, and that best moment linked to many more starting a year later.

Gratefulness.

Jennifer

As it grew closer and closer to late-July, I grew increasingly excited for camp at the Center For Courageous Kids again. It was going to be my second year, and I was happy to have the chance to see all of my friends again, most of which lived pretty far away. I hadn't seen ST in a whole year, which seemed like an impossibly long time.

My whole body bubbled with excitement as we neared Scottsville, Kentucky. In total, the drive had been a little over eight hours long, which we'd split between two different days. I looked out the window and saw a familiar winding road, which I knew led right to the camp. We were getting close!

A big sign featuring a giant lion dressed in scrubs came into view. CCK's mascot. We were here.

After we checked in, we found out we would be staying in the Blue Lodge that week. We immediately headed over to our cabin and brought our luggage over to our room.

We're here! I texted to Sarah Todd as soon as I sat down on my bed in our room, my unopened suitcase at my feet.

You're there before us! That's surprising. What cabin?? She responded. I laughed a little bit at the first part of her message as I remembered how her family had arrived way earlier than us the previous year.

Blue! Our room looks just like last year's, I typed. Right as I hit "send," I heard a knock at the door.

I didn't recall anyone ever knocking on the door of our room at camp the year before, so I was a little confused. My dad stopped unpacking his suitcase and walked over to the front of the room to open the door.

"We have a package for Starzec," the guy at the door said. My dad took the small, brown box from the man and thanked him.

I was very intrigued. I had a suspicion of what that box held, but I couldn't be completely sure yet.

I walked over to my dad's bed where he was ripping the packaging tape off of the box. As he did, I stole a glance at the shipping label and saw the word "Lulu." My suspicions grew even stronger.

"It's your book!" my dad exclaimed as he pulled it out of the box. I smiled as he handed it to me and immediately began leafing through it. It looked even better than I had expected! Even though we were already at the Center for Courageous

Kids, I grew even more jittery with anticipation than I'd been in the car on the way there, as I couldn't wait for ST to arrive so I could present her with our work.

My dad and siblings finished unpacking first, so the six of them left to go to the gym. The little kids were in desperate need of letting go of the energy that had built up during the long car ride, and the gym was a great place for that.

My book sat on top of the dresser next to my bed as I pulled clothes out of my bags and placed them into the drawers. Finally, my suitcase was completely empty. I looked over at my mom and saw that she was finished unpacking as well.

We left the blue cabin and started walking towards the gym, the book gripped tightly in my hand the whole time. When we walked past the Yellow Lodge, I noticed that Sadie—a seven -year-old with TM whom I'd met the year before—was playing outside of it with her siblings.

"Hey, Lisa! Hi, Jen!" Sadie's mom yelled to us as we approached. We greeted her as well, and she and my mom began talking. She asked me all of the usual adult-questions, and I responded appropriately, but was distracted the entire time; I couldn't stop myself from looking around for ST.

Just as I was thinking I must've missed her or that she was going to be hours late, I spotted a gray minivan drive up to the Red Lodge. Four people jumped out of the car before it drove away again to be parked, and I saw a familiar blonde ponytail amongst them.

I quickly excused myself from the conversation with my mom and Sadie's mom, and I started sprinting towards Red Lodge.

"SARAH TODD! ST! HAMMER!" I shouted, trying to catch her attention. Unfortunately, I was too far away; the family walked through the cabin's front doors, oblivious to my presence.

I slowed down to a fast walk, catching my breath. However, once I neared the cabin, I began running again. Finally, I reached the front entrance of the Red Lodge. I pulled open the heavy doors and slipped inside, still jogging.

"Jen?" I heard a deep voice say from behind me. I stopped and turned around to see ST's dad walking in, holding a couple suitcases.

"Hey," I said, completely out of breath. "Where's Sarah Todd? I wanted to show her this."

I held the book up for him to see, and he nodded before leading the way to the Hammers' assigned room.

We walked into the room, and I spotted Sarah Todd right away. She glanced up at the door and grinned when she spotted me.

"Jen!" she exclaimed, running up to hug me. I hugged her back, so excited to finally see my friend again. She was still significantly smaller than me, but 11-year-old ST definitely looked older and more mature than ten-year-old ST.

"Our book came!" I said as I handed the book to my co-author. She grabbed it and immediately started turning the pages.

"This is so cool!" She exclaimed.

~~~~~

"In a few minutes, they want all of the kids with TM to go to one of the rooms in there for a meeting," my mom said after lunch one day, pointing to one of the buildings in the circle of cabins that made up most of CCK. I had never been inside that particular cabin before, but I wasn't very excited to have a meeting with what I presumed would be a bunch of doctors.

"Do we have to? Can't we just hang out in the room?" ST whined beside me, likely feeling the same as I was. I nodded in agreement.

"Yes, you have to! They want everyone to go to this meeting. They're having one for the siblings, too, and I'm making your brothers go," Sarah Todd's mom said. My friend groaned and muttered something under her breath. I couldn't hear what she said, but it was probably a remark of protest.

"Come on," our moms said, leading the way to the front of the doctor-filled cabin. Sarah Todd and I looked at each other and sighed but grudgingly followed them.

As the four of us entered the building, a burst of cold air hit me. The AC seemed to always be blasting throughout every cabin at CCK, and this one was no exception.

Our moms left, and a counselor approached us by the entrance. He then led us to a decent-sized conference room where a bunch of other campers with TM sat. I found an empty chair next to a boy who looked to be around 11 or 12, and Sarah Todd sat across from me.

After a bunch of adults filed into the room and found seats at the head of the table, the meeting began.

During the meeting, we mostly did a lot of talking. The doctors gave us questions to discuss, beginning with fun, non-TM ones to break the ice, such as asking our favorite color and what job we wanted to pursue in the future. Afterwards, we moved on to questions about our experiences with Transverse Myelitis, and it was clear from the start that our stories were all vastly different.

Some kids talked about how they explained TM to other people and how the explanations were different when talking to little kids, peers, and adults. Some also spoke about some of their struggles with TM and whether other kids at school reacted to it by helping and being supportive or by bullying.

In the end, I felt as though I'd learned a lot about my fellow TMers, and though it pained me to admit it, I was glad I attended.

~~~~~

A day or two later, we were back in that same conference room-building. However, this time the doctors pulled us into individual rooms. ST and I had to wait near the front entrance for a few minutes after arriving at that building, but finally, my name was called. I waved to my friend, telling her to meet me in that same spot after we finished.

I followed the doctor into a small room, much smaller than the conference room the meeting had been in. I sat down, and he handed me a packet and a pencil.

"This is a test that asks questions concerning your mental state. We are using these in our research about how TM affects patients' minds. Your parents have signed a waiver that gives us permission to use your results in our studies. It will all be anonymous. You can withdraw your results from the study if you choose to do so," the man said after he sat down in front of me. I nodded and began filling my personal information in the front of the packet.

I flipped the page after all of that was recorded and started on the first question.

Immediately, I could tell that this was nothing new. I had taken pretty much the exact same test a couple times before when I had my neuropsychological tests done.

Some of the questions seemed ridiculous, and it seemed as though the same question was repeated a few times, just worded a bit differently each time. In the end, it didn't take all that long and wasn't too bad.

I handed him the packet, and he thanked me. Then, we proceeded to the next part, which was basically an incredibly shortened version of the neuropsych tests that I had suffered through twice before, both at Johns Hopkins and UT-Southwestern. He recorded my scores, and finally, I was able to go.

The tests were significantly shorter and less terrible than I'd imagined, but still, I was ready to leave the place and continue doing normal camp activities.

I walked over to the front entrance and sat down on one of the chairs there to wait for Sarah Todd to finish.

"Hey, Jen! Weren't those tests so annoying?"

Relief washed over me when Sarah Todd came into view. I grew even more relieved when our moms appeared behind the front doors to pick us up.

We left the cold building and entered the hot, humid Kentucky-air. Though that heat could be painful, right now it felt nice after hours in those freezing rooms.

I was happy to participate in those studies and greatly hoped the results from today would help them understand my condition a little better. I knew that scientists and doctors had only barely explored the surface of Transverse Myelitis and related illnesses and that they still had a long ways to go before getting to the point of understanding everything there is to know about them.

The more researchers learned about TM, ADEM, NMO, AFM, etc., the more they'd be able to understand it. And I knew that the more they understood it, the better they could figure out what causes it and how to treat it, amongst other things.

Sarah Todd and I lagged behind our moms a bit and chatted. We reached the dining hall for dinner and were immediately greeted with music and energy. I looked around and smiled at all of the kids who were so excited to be at camp and see their friends—friends they'd likely keep in touch with the rest of their lives. Hanging out with others with TM taught us so much; although no two people are affected by this condition in the exact same way, TM friends can still relate to so many things—things that our other friends back home would likely never be able to come close to understanding.

And for all of that, I was incredibly grateful. If this disease had to make an appearance in my life, at least it brought these people with it.

Enjoyment.

Sarah Todd

I couldn't wait to go to CCK for the second time in July. Jen was going, our first book had just been published, I had choreographed dances I wanted to show Jen, and she wanted to record them. I was a bit bummed when we arrived at camp and found out we were in the red lodge because I had previously texted Jen, and she was in the blue lodge. Although we weren't in the same lodge, and I was a little bummed, we still had our activities together, so we got lucky with our lodge placements.

Eagerly sitting on my bed in our den, I felt jumpy and excited because I couldn't wait to see our book. To my luck, after waiting just a few minutes, Jen came in carrying *5k, Ballet, and a Spinal Cord Injury*. First, I hugged her, and she handed me the book with a huge smile on her face. We both jumped on my bed, opening the book and perusing through it. I turned to the epilogue, and Jen laughed. Turning to her, I asked her what was so funny.

"It actually says 'prologue' instead of 'epilogue.' My dad's going to fix it," she said, and I couldn't help but think that was pretty funny. *Good thing no one bought the book yet*, I thought. We didn't have enough books at camp to do a book signing/selling, so we made flyers that we signed, planning to hand them out to everyone.

Aside from all the stuff we wanted to do to promote our book, Jen also really wanted to film me performing my many dances I had choreographed. Over FaceTime that summer, we put together a costume (which was just clothes from my dresser) for each dance, and I brought all of them to camp. We made a list of my dances and their recording order, which was: *Sarah Todd's Dances*: *La Creme De La Creme*, *Silver Spoons*, *Cry*, *I Want It Now*, *Beautiful Day*, *Describing the Car Crash*, *Girls in the House*, *and That's Where It Is*. Before TM, I had never thought about choreographing a dance. But, after I started watching *Dance Moms* in 2012, I thought it'd be fun to try choreographing dances to some of the songs from the show. This was one of the best decisions I ever made because I helped myself find a new hobby formed from my original one.

For my dance videos, I needed a place with plenty of empty space and where people hardly passed by. After searching all throughout the camp for the appropriate spot to record, Jen and I settled in an open space right outside our favorite place: the gym. Even though nobody was around when we arrived, I was nervous somebody would walk in and see me dancing. It seems silly, but ever since I started dancing to my DVDs in my family room at home, I never wanted anyone watching me unless I had specifically prepared a certain dance and invited people to watch. The stage felt much more comfortable than my own house—it was my second home.

~~~~~

Arts and crafts weren't mine and Jen's favorite thing to do because of TM, for sure, but we figured we could create something cool if we helped each other. We sat with our favorite counselor, Amanda, and she helped us paint wooden mustaches, then add sparkles on them. I painted mine black and covered it in pink, purple, and silver sparkles, and Jen painted hers yellow and covered it in silver sparkles. After we decorated the mustaches, we glued popsicle sticks on them so we could hold them up to our faces, and we took lots of pictures with them.

Even though making the mustaches was fun, we couldn't wait to continue on to one of our most favorite camp activities: swimming. A large, unoccupied float sat on one side of the pool, so we swam and grabbed it. Thinking it'd be fun, we both climbed on the float at the same time to see if we'd both fit, and the float toppled over, sending us underwater. I was thankful the water wasn't crazy deep, I didn't back-flip, and I had the capability to pull my head out of the water safely, back on my feet. Laughing, we tried again, but this time, Jen got on first and helped me balance on the float. Once we were successful, we floated around the pool until our arms got tired of pushing us.

~~~~~

Many different hospitals and doctors were constantly doing research studies on people with TM and their siblings to compare different things. I had participated in several at a few places because I wanted to help, although they were never very fun. Jen and I were hanging out in the dining hall when a woman approached us asking if we'd be willing to participate in a study for TM patients and siblings testing reaction time, memory, and brain-fog on iPads. For an unknown reason, some people with TM have delayed reaction time, not as good of a memory, and brain fog. I was fortunate enough to not have any of these, but I knew my results would be important to their study, so I agreed, as did Jen. On our way to the medical building, I turned to Jen and joked, "She probably thought we're siblings since we look like we don't have TM."

~~~~

Around the third day of camp, two paralympians with TM spoke about their wheelchair sports and what someone would need to do to begin training to compete in the Paralympics. One of the women did wheelchair racing, and the other one did adaptive skiing. Throughout their speeches, they gave a lot of helpful tips for anyone who might've wanted to try either of their sports.

A few of my friends were interested, I thought, but Jen and I weren't. For one thing, I've never been a sporty girl; the closest I ever got to doing a sport was cheering, and I never planned to do anything closer than that. And, for another thing, the paralympics were mostly aimed for people in wheelchairs.

~~~~~

During the morning before everyone was going to leave, the talent show took place, which I knew Jen and a lot of other people wished I was performing in, but I made that my goal for next time. I knew I'd be better prepared and extremely ready to perform in the talent show next year—I wasn't going to miss my opportunity. Jen and I hugged tightly as we left, as always, and I promised myself I'd perform on that stage in a year.

Commitment.

Jennifer

Every year, the cross country coaches took the top ten boys and top ten girls on the team to a huge meet all the way in Peoria, Illinois, which was about three hours away. They took two of our school's big vans down there the day before the meet and stayed in a hotel that night.

Freshman year, I had actually been pretty close to making the top ten, but not quite. I wasn't disappointed at all that year though; I was pretty sure I would eventually have the chance to go in the future, most likely as an upperclassman.

However, the opportunity ended up being closer than I'd anticipated. I was now a sophomore, and when Coach informed me that I was one of the top ten girls on the team, I was ecstatic. It was also a little hard to believe! I had worked really hard and had a lot of goals in cross country—such as making Varsity by junior year —and now that I was in the top ten, those goals felt even more attainable. It may not seem like a huge deal to some, but it felt like a pretty big one to me; I was excited.

The three-hour drive down to Peoria was very interesting. My back was killing me the entire time, for one thing, though that didn't come as a big surprise. I had a pillow behind it, but it only helped for so long; my back usually hurt after just a few minutes of sitting up. Luckily, though, I was very distracted; the senior girls were dancing and singing crazily, which I found very funny and entertaining. After they quieted down a little, everyone somehow simultaneously decided to take a nap. By the time most of us woke up, we were nearly at our destination.

~~~~~

As my teammates and I stood at the starting line the next morning, I noticed just how enormous the race was. The line of girls stretched really far on either side of me; I couldn't believe I was going to be racing against all of them!

They were probably all really good, too. And much faster than you.

I tried to push those thoughts away, but I was really anxious. I knew that there was no way I was the slowest girl there and that place didn't matter at all. Time didn't even matter a whole lot either, honestly. I always tried to run my fastest and improve my personal record, but the most important thing was to enjoy myself and the experience.

The race began, and all of the girls in that gigantic crowd were off. Unfortunately, I immediately got stuck behind some people, which grew annoying; there were so many runners and so little space on the course that I couldn't get in front of them. After trying and failing to squeeze through the thick group of girls right ahead of me, I relented and fell into a slower pace behind them. Occasionally I'd find a little opening and manage to speed up a little bit more, but in general, I was unable to get to the pace where I wanted to be. I quickly decided that I much preferred the more medium-sized races where I could still weave between other runners to get ahead.

I ended up finishing with a pretty decent time. I hadn't been running as slow as I'd thought, but I wasn't even close to beating my personal record. However, I couldn't deny that it had been a good experience. The weather had been nice; sunny —but not too hot—and not insanely humid. Though I wasn't in love with that course or the race itself, the whole thing was a good experience, and I was still very excited to be on the top ten. I couldn't wait to see what was coming for me next.

~~~~~

After the enormity of the Top Ten meet, I couldn't wait to get back to the normal races closer to home that I was more used to.

Not too long afterwards, it came time for my favorite meet again. This one had the best course and was the meet I'd gotten my huge personal record—22:45— freshman year. It seemed as if the weather and everything was going to be very similar to the year before, and I was very excited for the conditions to repeat themselves. I wasn't expecting another huge personal record, especially since I had yet to beat 22:45 in the past year, but I still hoped for it in the back of my mind.

When the race started, I tried to begin a little slower, just like I'd done on that course the year before. I really, really wanted to experience that race again, as it had been one of the best days of my life! Or the best 22 minutes and 45 seconds of my life, anyway. But after running for a few minutes, I gave up; I knew it was impossible, and my best bet was to just run it without overthinking every step.

It didn't go nearly as smoothly as the 22:45-race; my legs felt like they were working much harder, and I didn't have last year's seniors' energetic cheering to distract me. However, I still felt like I was doing pretty well. I seemed to be passing a lot of people, and I was able to speed up quite a bit during the last mile.

"Keep it up, J-Star!" Coach cheered as I passed by him. I smiled, remembering how he'd cheered me on from the exact same spot in the woods the year before. Then I remembered what he'd said to me from that spot the year before: *If you're smiling, you're not running fast enough.*

I shifted my focus back to the race and realized that it was somehow almost over. I felt like I'd only finished one mile, not three; just like the same race the year before, this one had flown by.

Naturally, I sprinted to the finish line as soon as I saw it. As I slowed to a stop, I caught sight of the clock.

21:45.

I shaved exactly one minute off of last year's time.

That may not seem like much to some people, but to runners, even a ten-second improvement is huge! Even though the 22:45-race would always hold a special place in my heart, I was proud of myself and very excited about my new personal record.

I even got a medal, which I hung on my bedroom wall as soon as I got home.

Confidence.

Sarah Todd

Sadly, summer had to come to an end at some point, and in 2013, summer ending meant middle school for me. Every year, I was pretty excited for a new school year because summer got boring after three months. However, in 2013, I was terrified for school to start for obvious reasons. Clearly, the main reason was that I was going to attend a brand new school with only about twenty people from my elementary school coming with me. Twenty kids sounded like quite a bit, but when there were 450 students in each grade, there wasn't much of a chance I'd know someone in each of my classes.

Even though I was worried about friends, I didn't have to worry as much about getting to know my teachers because I attended a meeting with all my teachers for the whole school year a few weeks before school began. In the meeting, I learned my class schedule for First Quarter, and all the teachers introduced themselves and told me what they taught. Having the meeting helped me to be less nervous for the start of school since I somewhat knew my teachers and they knew all about me and my accommodations.

In addition to the school meeting, one of the employees at my new school took me on a tour of the entire place so I could see what my surroundings were like. During my tour, I tried opening doors to the front office, all my potential classrooms, and the clinic. I struggled to open some of the doors, so I remembered which ones they were so I could ask for help with them and be independent on the doors I knew I could handle. Then, I picked my locker, which was a bottom one on the end so I could reach it easily and not get stuck in the huge crowd of students. Plus, the locker above mine was left vacant so that I wouldn't accidentally get hit with books or the locker door. We also decided that it'd be easier for me to bring my own lunch instead of buy one every day so that I wouldn't have to deal with the huge crowds in the cafeteria.

Getting to tour the school made me excited and took some of the nerves away, and I knew I'd adjust to middle school in no time—I just had a little extra to worry about and deal with than most other kids starting middle school.

In sixth grade, I still had an assistant. Having an adult constantly attached to my hip wasn't ideal, but since I didn't know if I'd have a friend I already knew in each of my classes that may be able to help me, the school decided it'd be better for me to have an assistant once again. The school found an assistant for me, but something happened, and she had to move. So, I didn't get to meet the new assistant until the third day of school, which upset me a little since I wanted to be able to get to know her right away instead of having a substitute the first couple of days. But, everything turned out fine, as I knew it would. Of course, I wasn't thrilled about having an assistant at all; I wanted to be a normal sixth grader, and I couldn't be normal if I had an adult following me around at all times. Though, I had learned quickly that life doesn't always go the way I want it to, and that's okay. I still plod on.

~~~~~

My assistant and I quickly came up with a routine every morning: we'd go into my homeroom, which was the first classroom in the sixth grade hall, and put my lunchbox on the counter. I didn't have homeroom first period—I had it third with lunch—so there'd always be some kids I didn't know in the classroom waiting for their first class to start. After stopping in my homeroom, I'd go to the bathroom while she grabbed my supplies from my locker so I could avoid the crowd of kids.

One thing I hadn't thought about was that at my elementary school, most of my friends got the gist of what had happened to me because we had been in school together, and my mom came in and spoke to my class in fourth grade about what had happened to me. But, in my new middle school, most people didn't know anything about me, let alone my disability. Having to explain my situation to my new friends, answer classmate's questions, and receive odd looks from other students made me a little apprehensive, but I knew I would find a good response to everything asked, said, and done as time went on.

Every morning I couldn't help but notice that when my assistant went to put my lunchbox down while I stood by the door waiting for her, the kids in the room would stare at me. I knew for sure that they were wondering why I had an adult following me around all day, because I knew I'd be curious as well if I were they. The stares were annoying, but I knew they didn't mean any harm. So, every morning, smiling at them became part of my routine, too.

I made friends quickly, most of them being in my homeroom. We had lunch together, so we were able to get to know one another well. Constantly getting asked questions about things that were different for me was tiring, so I wanted to tell my friends about TM as soon as possible. But, finding a good time to tell them and a good way to do it without it being slightly awkward and filled with mumbled "that's awful" and "I'm so sorry"s proved to be difficult.

~~~~~

The whole sixth grade had to take a standardized test at the beginning of the school year, and I was allowed to complete mine online so I wouldn't have to spend time I didn't have bubbling in my answers. Before the test, I saw a friend in the hall.

"Where are you going?"

"I'm taking my test in the computer lab," I explained to her, knowing she'd ask why.

Here it comes... "Why?"

"I need extra time," I answered simply, trying not to make it a big deal.

She replied with an "okay" and a smile—no questions, no remarks about how "lucky" I was to be eligible for extra time... Why was I so worried about telling them?

The test encounter gave me the perfect excuse to explain myself. So, I told my new, small group of friends about TM, and whenever I needed help with anything, they were happy to help me. Since I began to be able to trust my friends and rely on them to help me, I found myself not needing my assistant's help as much. This made me extremely happy because having my friends help me was way more normal and didn't attract as much attention to myself.

After telling my new friends about TM, I was so relieved that I didn't have to worry about giving an explanation anymore. To others, it probably seems as if something as trivial as this shouldn't make me so anxious, but it did; I don't like feeling as if I can't ask someone for help because I'm afraid they'll wonder why I'd need help with something "everyone can do." Eventually, my friends learned what I needed help with, and I didn't even have to ask them every time I needed something anymore, which made me thankful I made such lovely friends.

Perseverance.

Jennifer

"We have to get up and get ready," I whispered, shaking my friend. She groaned, but after I continuously poked her, she eventually complied.

It was still pitch-black outside, which meant it was a time of morning that we *really* did not want to be awake for, but we had to be up this early today because we were going to help out at one of the water stations at the Chicago Half Marathon. I knew it was going to be fun, but I was definitely tired. However, we got lucky that my aunt had let my friend, my mom, and me sleep at her house that night; she lived way closer to where the race was taking place than we did. If we had departed from our house, we probably would've had to wake up an hour earlier.

By the time we arrived at the water station where we'd volunteer, the sky was beginning to show the faintest strokes of morning; the black was slowly being replaced by pale reds, oranges, and yellows. I was rarely awake to see the sunrise, so I appreciated being able to see it.

As soon as we walked over to the tables, a lady gave each of us a yellow t-shirt that identified us as volunteers before instructing us on what to do.

Some of the tables at our station were going to have cups of Gatorade, while the others would have cups of water. I watched while a few people poured water into big containers from the many water jugs they had out. Then, we poured Gatorade concentrate into the containers and mixed it with the water really well.

Next, we set paper cups out on the tables before pouring either Gatorade or water into them. Boards went on top of each row of cups so they could be stacked high on top of each other as well, and by the end, each table held a *lot* of paper cups. Of course, there were also going to be a lot of people in the race, most of which would likely need hydration.

In front of our water station was a road—which was where people were going to be running—and on the other side of that road was a long, metal rail that looked over some other streets below, which was where some of the beginning of the race was going to take place. After we finished setting everything up, a lot of us walked over to that rail so we could watch the runners below; our water station was closer to the finish line, so we wouldn't have anyone near us for a while, but we knew the half marathon was starting very soon.

The first people we saw were wheelchair racers, who seemed to be going incredibly fast. I was immediately reminded of the ladies who had spoken to us at camp that past July, because one of them had talked a bit about wheelchair racing. The chairs didn't look comfortable at all, and it seemed like they took a lot of arm strength; however, I admired those people and was glad that racing was an option available to them. While watching them, I couldn't help but wonder about all of those people's stories. Were they lost for a while before discovering that they could try this sport and realized they loved it and excelled at it? I knew a few people like that, who were unable to get back to a sport they loved pre-disability, but instead discovered their passion for a different hobby or an adaptive sport afterwards. I didn't really know what that was like; I'd felt a little lost before recovering enough to run again after TM, but that was quickly resolved after I was able to get back to my sport, and I already knew that I loved running. The sport I loved most wasn't something I discovered post-disability, and I wondered a little bit about what that might be like.

~~~~~

When the runners finally approached our station, we stood by the tables with cups in hand, ready for them to be snatched as they passed us. However, that was not the case for the first few runners. They were the ones who had times and people to beat, so they were going really, really fast; apparently, they did not want to be slowed down by getting water at every station.

More fast runners came next, but they weren't quite as crazy-fast as the first few. Most of these ones took water and/or Gatorade, but they were still going fast as they grabbed the cups from volunteers, splashing a lot of us in the process. They didn't seem to slow down much to drink it either; for the most part, they seemed to throw the liquid at their faces and hope for the best. I couldn't imagine they got more than a few drops inside their mouths, but I suppose that could be better than nothing.

After that, the stream of runners gradually thickened. By the time the runners with more average paces got to us, it was hectic. It was a long, thick group, and the vast majority of them wanted water. I handed one water cup after another, and everyone else around me did the same. I was definitely a little bit slower than most of the other volunteers because they were able to easily hand cups out with both hands; when I tried holding cups out in my right hand, I ended up dropping a few, spilling water at people's feet. However, in general, I was still able to successfully give water to a lot of runners.

The stream of racers eventually thinned out again, until no one remained on the road in front of us. By now, the sun was blazing down on us, and everyone was completely worn out. However, it was a very rewarding experience. The longest races I'd run so far in my life were only 3.1 miles, but seeing all of the people in this race made me very excited for the future. At this point, I didn't know when I'd have the chance to run a half-marathon, but I hoped to sometime soon.

Wisdom.

Sarah Todd

"You're so lucky!" one of my friends said to me as my teacher went and grabbed a chair for me to sit in while everyone else sat on the floor.

"Why?" I asked her. "Because I get to sit in a chair?"

"Yeah! I hate sitting on the floor," she expressed dramatically.

My teacher came back with my chair and put it in the circle where everyone else was sitting. When I sat down, I felt like I was standing out more than everyone else because I was up higher, which I didn't like at all, although I knew I couldn't sit on the floor and hurt my tailbone and neck. I so desperately wanted to ask my classmate if she would rather be allowed to sit in a chair instead of on the floor or if she'd rather have the use of her arms and hands. But, I knew I couldn't do that, so I ended up not saying anything. She would get over it eventually.

~~~~~

"Sarah Todd is so lucky; I wish I was her," another one of my classmates said randomly during social studies one day.

"Why?" my teacher asked her.

176

"Well, because. She didn't have to take the CRCT exam," she complained.

My teacher responded, "Yes, she did. She took it last year—just not with our class."

"Oh."

~~~~~

I had an essay to write for English, and I didn't want my hand to get tired. So, my assistant brought out my netbook computer my school provided for me so that I could complete my work.

"I wish I had a computer," the boy next to me exclaimed.

"Why?" I asked. "It's a pain having to get it out and set it up."

"Because, spell check is on there! You don't have to worry about misspelling anything, and you can cheat," he whined.

"My spell check is turned off," I explained, "so I can't cheat… not that I ever would."

"Oh, that stinks."

~~~~~

"You're so lucky! You get extra time on the exam," yet another classmate said to me.

"Yeah, well, my hand gets tired easily, so I need more time to write," I tried to explain to her.

~~~~~

"Can you open my candy for me, please?" I asked a friend.

"Sure! Only if I can have some, though."

So my choices are to either share some even though I'm very hungry, or not have my candy opened at all.

~~~~~

Every day, everyone faces their own struggles. My biggest struggles most days are, of course, my arm paralysis and needing a lot of extra help to do certain things. Most people with disabilities, chronic illnesses, etc. need more assistance and get more "benefits" than the average person just to help us get through our days.

When able-bodied people tell me that I'm lucky because I receive these "benefits" (things such as extra time on tests or getting to type certain things), it's insulting. I know that some people have good intentions and are just trying to understand what I'm dealing with, or they're trying to point out the "positives" (as if I don't already know them), but it never works that way. In that case, it's invasive and not necessary. In most cases, though, they truly are jealous of the "benefits" I receive and clearly disregard the fact that my hands and arms don't work as they should. I need that extra assistance and "benefits," because they help me get through my days without as much of a hassle.

We disabled people aren't different from anybody else; we just need extra help —whether it be hands, wheels, equipment, or simple adaptations—to make life easier. Some able-bodied people go as far as to say they'd like to be in a wheelchair for a day because it seems "fun." The truth to that, though, is that it's only "fun" if you can get out of that chair.

~~~~~

Most people are too nervous to ask me what happened or why I need help with certain things, but as long as I'm asked nicely and I'll be seeing the person a lot (so it'd be helpful for them to know), I don't mind at all! No one understands how great it feels to have the weight off my shoulders after a new friend asks questions—it feels great. It feels great knowing they won't be curious anymore. It feels great knowing they're someone I can ask for help. And, it feels great knowing they're trying to understand and be a good friend. Support feels great, and I hope I'll receive it no matter where I go.

Motivation.

Jennifer

It was October 6th, 2013, and I was on my way to Illinois' first ever Walk-Run-N-Roll for Transverse Myelitis.

The park that the event was taking place at was about an hour away from my house. Registration was starting at ten, but my family had agreed to be there early to help out, so we departed at around eight that morning.

A couple of my friends—Grace and Val—had decided that they wanted to join us at the walk, so my mom drove the three of us while my dad and siblings went separately in our big car.

Over and over again, I read the sticky-notes that I had stuck to my copy of *5k, Ballet, and a Spinal Cord Injury*. I had been asked to speak about my story and book at the walk, so the night before, I had spent a couple hours trying to pick the perfect passages to read and attempting to write the perfect introduction. I wasn't completely satisfied with what I'd come up with, but it was good enough.

Before I knew it, we had arrived. When we walked towards the park from the parking lot, the first thing I noticed was that a bunch of sports wheelchairs sat next to the basketball court. Some other people were already there, and I saw that a few kids—some with TM, some able-bodied—were playing basketball in those sports wheelchairs. My siblings immediately ran over to join them while the rest of us helped set up.

I was directed to a folding table where I could sign and sell my books. It was across from the tables holding the raffle and auction items and next to another folding table where a man seemed to be selling or giving away some things.

My dad took a box of books out of the car and placed it under the table. I took a few out of the box and laid them neatly on the tabletop so people could see what they looked like and read the summary on the back. I then set out the metal money box we'd brought as well, and in front of it, I placed a stack of mini-flyers that explained our book and listed our website and where to buy it, in case people didn't have money on them today but wanted to get one later.

I sat down behind the table when I was finished and watched as a bunch of people came to the park. The day wasn't terribly cold, but it wasn't particularly warm, either; a breeze went by, and I shivered a bit in my sweatshirt.

After everyone was done with registration and everything, the walk/run/roll was able to begin. First, they called everyone over for some pictures with the huge sign that read "2013 Illinois Walk-Run-N-Roll for TMA." They took a couple pictures of everyone there, as well as a couple of just the people with TM. After that was done, they let us start on the course.

Although it was less than two miles, it wasn't going to be timed, and there weren't going to be any first place medals at the end, Grace was competitive and wanted us to try to "win." So, we ran the whole thing, leaving the majority of the group way behind us.

"We're ahead of everyone!" Grace exclaimed.

"Yeah. We had a lot of competition. The lady pushing that stroller almost beat us," I responded sarcastically.

"Actually, we're not the first ones," Val said, pointing out a group of little boys cutting across the grass in front of us.

"That doesn't count! They're cheating!" Grace screeched dramatically.

We continued running and made it to the finish in barely any time at all. A lady handed us each a participation medal.

"See?" Grace said, holding her medal up. "We *did* win first place."

~~~~~

A lot of people spoke about TM and different TM-related things after everyone had completed the walk. I sat at my little table next to my friends, trying to pay attention to what they were saying but way too nervous to focus on anything other than the panic and anxiety that public speaking always stirred up.

"Our next speaker is Jen Starzec! She is 15 and is going to talk a little bit about about her experiences with TM, as well as the book she and a friend wrote about it."

182

I was startled when I heard my name coming from the other side of the gazebo we were in, so I hesitated. Slowly, I stood up and made my way to the front.

"Um... Hi, I'm Jen," I stuttered awkwardly, wincing as I heard my voice amplified by the microphone. I looked down at my book and started reading off the sticky-notes.

I tried not to look down the whole time, knowing that it was best to glance up frequently when reading something in front of people, but it was much easier to avoid seeing the crowd's expectant gazes pointed right at me.

After I finished my introduction, I read the passages I'd bookmarked. I stumbled over the words a few times, mentally hitting myself each time since I literally wrote them myself. Finally, I was done, and I scurried back to my table as quickly as I could, my face red-hot with embarrassment.

"I was way too quiet. That was so awkward," I mumbled to my friends and family after I sat down. Of course, they assured me that I did well, but I didn't quite believe them.

However, my speaking must have piqued the interest of at least a portion of the crowd, because at the end of the event, a lot of people came up to me to buy books or take flyers. Many of them asked me questions and told me I did well, too. I still thought I had been really awkward up there, but I at least started to feel like I didn't do horrendously.

As we drove away from that park when the event was over and headed towards home, I couldn't help but be really happy about how the day had turned out. We had succeeded in raising a ton of money for the Transverse Myelitis Association, which was always a great thing. And, even though I didn't thoroughly enjoy speaking in front of everyone, I knew it was a good experience for me, and I had a ton of fun overall.

I couldn't wait to see what would happen at the Walk-Run-N-Roll next year.

Part III:

2014

As they progressed in their recoveries,
Finding new, different ways to do things,
Everyone beamed at their discoveries.
Though they do not know what the future brings,
One runs with vigor, one dances with grace.
They talk every day, all laughs, cheers, and smiles—
Neither wants those memories to efface.
They're separated by thousands of miles;
Two cities never seemed so far away.
Greatly missing each other endlessly,
They know their bond as friends will always stay.
If one has feelings of disparity,
The other will come running to their side,
And they will be thankful their best friend tried.

Poem by Sarah Todd Hammer

Dreams.

Sarah Todd

Sometimes, when Jen and I are a bit bored and texting about nothing in particular, we ask each other questions about TM, which is a topic we usually stray away from. Even though it's not our favorite subject, it's always a relief knowing that someone who understands is there to talk and vent to. I know at least trying to understand what happened to our bodies and what's happening to them now is important because it's necessary to be informed and knowledgeable, and I *want* to be informed and knowledgeable.

"If you woke up and didn't have TM, what would you do the whole day?" Jen asked me. I contemplated my answer for a second, going through my days *with* TM in my head, thinking of all the things I would love to do normally again—even if it was just for one day.

"I'd get up, shower, brush my teeth, do my makeup, get dressed, tie my shoes…" I stopped typing, thinking about how crazy it was that I wished to do all these daily tasks that most people do without paying any attention to them at all.

I imagined myself tying my own shoes and smiled. Then I realized, though, that I didn't remember how to tie my shoes. Usually, I wore shoes like flip flops or sandals so I could put them on without help, but occasionally, I'd have to wear tennis shoes. Because I hadn't tied my shoes independently since getting TM, the steps were no longer imprinted in my brain. This disappointed me because I'd learned how to tie my shoes early—when I was about four—and here I was, 13 years old, and unable to tie my shoes. When a necessity is taken away, it becomes a want. And, I had learned that quickly.

Gathering my thoughts again, I added, "run downstairs, open the fridge, grab any food I usually can't open, open it, scoop my own ice cream, open the heaviest doors in the house, reach for anything up high, put my backpack on and off, dance doing all the arm movements, a cartwheel, swim, type with both hands, hold things I normally wouldn't with my left hand, probably shower again, and go to sleep."

I sent her my answer then asked, "What would you do?"

She answered with, "I'd wake up early, go on a long run, do arm exercises, shower, dry and straighten my hair, cartwheels and handstands, hangout with my friends, play the piano, write with my right hand, and fall asleep easily."

It was interesting to see the differences in our answers; there were some things she'd wish to do on a day without TM that I hadn't thought of. Every activity we wanted to do was something that seemed trivial, but they can be compared to not seeing a friend for a long time: someone has a best friend, and they're inseperable, but they have to move away. The person immediately realizes how much they'll miss their best friend and that they took their close proximity for granted. Now, whenever they see each other again, it's a blessing. Neither of us realized how much we loved being able to do "small," daily activities until they were taken away from us.

~~~~~

After watching *Soul Surfer* one time in Baltimore, I was inspired to start trying new things and find adaptive ways to do them. First, I started with tying my shoes. At KKI, I learned how to tie my shoes with one hand during OT. It took some fancy thinking on my OT's part to come up with a fairly easy way to do it, and learning how was quite frustrating. I had to place my other foot on the left lace and pull the right one with my right hand to get them tight. Then, I could cross the laces with my right hand, but they always became loose when I had to pull the lace under the 'x.' The 'bunny ears' gave me loads of trouble, and even after the numerous times I tried, the final product always turned out too loose, so I couldn't walk in the shoes anyway. Sometimes it just seemed easier to have someone help me do something if they were around, but sandals and flip flops still continued to be my best buddies.

Next, I moved on to making a PB&J, because PB&Js were one of my absolute favorite sandwiches, but making one wasn't as easy as I thought it'd be. I didn't think about how hard it would be to open the peanut butter and jelly jars or the bread, and I definitely didn't think spreading the peanut butter and jelly on the bread

192

would be *that* tedious. Mom opened the jars for me, but I opted to still try the rest, wanting to do most of the job. My final product was messy and didn't taste as good as Mom's PB&Js, but I was proud of myself anyway.

~~~~~

Annually, I have an MRI of my brain and cervical spine as a precaution to check on my spinal cord scarring and make sure nothing has changed. I always dread MRIs, particularly because mine are ordered with and without contrast, which means I need an IV. IVs shouldn't be a problem, and they haven't always been, but I had an awful experience once where the nurses attempted to insert the IV six times until they were victorious. Because of TM, I'm extremely sensitive to cooler temperatures, especially on my left side since it's flaccid. The IVs were difficult to put in because my arms and hands were so cold. So, whenever I need an MRI now, I opt to have the anesthesia through a mask instead of through the IV so that I'll be asleep while they put the IV in, which works way better. After one horrifying experience, I avoid IVs as much as possible. The mask is still scary, and the whole MRI ordeal is nerve-wracking, but any alternate solution to having an IV is worth it.

Aside from IVs being an issue, staying still for an MRI is hard for anyone to do, but it's especially hard after having TM. After not being able to move anything, I have to always be moving *some* part of my body—even if it means simply wiggling my toes. I can never stay completely still again.

"I will never tell her to 'be still' ever again," my mom says.

Goals.

Jennifer

"Let it goooo, let it goooo!" I sang at the top of my lungs. It was evening and pitch-black out. The only reason I could see anything at all was due to the faint moon and stars, as well as the few streetlights scattered across the neighborhood. Tonight, my friend Grace and I were running. We were training for the biggest race of our lives: a half marathon, or 13.1 miles of sheer self-inflicted torture. On this particular night, we were running nine miles, which was the most we'd run so far.

"Jen!" Grace screeched, cutting off my singing. "How do you have this much joy eight miles into a nine-mile run?!"

I laughed, but stopped belting Disney songs. The truth was, I had no idea where the happiness was coming from. I mean, I was extremely exhausted! But there was something about running in the dark when no one else was out and most houses were no longer lit up, their inhabitants likely asleep. There was something about the brisk, night-time air, which was perfect for running. There was something about being able to jog underneath the sliver of a moon and glittering stars, of being able to look up and see the Big Dipper and Orion, all in the same spot no matter how many miles we moved.

There was a time when I would have thought a half marathon an impossible goal. Actually, there were many times when it seemed that way. Even when I'd first signed up for the race and therefore dedicated myself to training for the thing, I'd had my doubts. But now, running nine miles—five more than I'd ever run before that spring—I knew it was close. That goal *was* possible, after all! I was going to run a half marathon.

As Grace and I slowed to a stop, finishing our run for the day, I thought about how hard we'd worked to get to that point. The training hadn't been easy; it really did seem like we were starting all the way at the bottom.

~~~~~

The half-marathon training journey began in late February or early March of 2014. A few of my friends signed up for it as well, and we were all extremely excited for the opportunity to say we were able to run 13.1 miles straight!

13.1 miles is an incredibly difficult goal for any able-bodied person, so I knew going into it that it would be even harder for me. However, I was determined to achieve the goals I'd set for myself back when I started running in sixth grade.

I told myself at age 11 or 12 that I was going to run a half marathon, full marathon, and triathlon when I was older. I didn't expect to be paralyzed—amongst other things—by a rare spinal cord-damaging condition just a year and a half or so later, of course. TM definitely complicated the possibility of those future plans. However, I also knew that I *could* run a half marathon if I really worked at it. I knew that I'd be wiped out for the rest of the day after every time I trained, and I knew that I'd likely be unable to get out of bed for a week after the race. I knew that my pain levels would be greatly heightened for awhile.

But I was too determined to let any of that stop me. I was determined to be able to cross one thing off that goal list I'd made for myself in sixth grade.

I wasn't going to let anything stop me from doing so.

Spirit.

Sarah Todd

After a few weeks of planning and coordinating with our moms, Jen had plane tickets from Chicago to Atlanta! The whole trip seemed to appear out of nowhere as it felt as if we were discussing it one moment, and the next, I was in my car with my parents going to pick Jen up from the airport. The whole day at school, I told my friends what was happening and how excited I was; it was a huge deal for her to have the opportunity to come all the way from Chicago! Jen and I were so excited once her plane tickets were bought that we could hardly mention the topic without squealing—*literally*. In order to help us contain our excitement and occupy our minds for the preceding 40 days, we each put 20 different activities in our notes on our phones; then, we ripped pieces of paper and numbered each piece from 1 to 20. Every day after school, we alternated and drew a number from the hat. After one of us drew the number, we looked in our notes on our phone and both of us did the designated activity for that number on FaceTime together.

Anyway, when my parents and I arrived at the "busiest airport in the world," we figured out which gate Jen's flight would be coming in on, and we took the train down there. I had envisioned Jen walking out the jetway while I waited for her to be close enough so we could hug and yell out our dumb and playful insult greetings we had planned beforehand, but as we approached her gate, she was nearly the last one sitting there. Despite our mild disappointment about her early flight (better early than late), we hugged tightly while my mom took pictures.

Neither of us know why, but whenever we haven't seen each other in several months, we feel awkward at first, and we think the other looks *so* much different that we *had* to have just hugged the wrong person… no, really. It's weird. The temporary awkwardness is especially unexplained and unfathomable because we can text each other whatever comes into our minds—be it serious, weird, funny, stupid, *whatever*—yet we feel as if we hardly know each other when we first see each other. But, that always changes within thirty minutes—*max*. It was gone as soon as we took weird selfies in the car.

I have always had an extreme love for the photobooth app, so we knew we just had to use it on my mac. She, my brother Alex, and I went crazy with the hilarious pictures we took for an hour, and we were laughing the whole time. Somehow, I never got sick of photobooth, and it made for a super fun activity to do Jen's first night here. Later that night (or morning since it was about one), we took my makeup from my vanity and did blind makeovers—the most typical sleepover activity for teenaged girls. I, at age 12, hadn't really worn makeup, but when I did, I wore tan eyeshadow and lip gloss, which I thought was super amazing and cool.

But, I've come to realize (thankfully) that if eyeshadow is applied, mascara should

be, too. Although, by the end of each of our blind makeovers, I had lip gloss on my

nose, and Jen had bright, pink lipstick on her forehead. From the get-go we knew

our makeovers were going to be horrendous—what, with our partially paralyzed

hands and all—but they were super fun to attempt.

~~~~~

I knew for awhile then that I was going to choreograph a dance to "Falling

Slowly" from *Once* since I recently watched the movie, but I hadn't started on it yet.

So, as if the blind makeovers weren't enough for the approaching dawn, Jen filmed

me improvising to the song to compare with how the actual dance would eventually

turn out when I was finished choreographing it. My jetés were looking really good

(especially my left one), and I incorporated a few of those into my improv because I

always wanted my strongest points to stand out in my dances. By the last short

video we filmed, though, I was extremely tired given the time and all my exercise,

and my feet became so floppy they looked like fish on a dock.

A couple days later, when I had gained plenty of energy back, Jen showed me a

great song she found on YouTube called "Heart" that she thought would be an

excellent song to choreograph a dance to. The song was dedicated to tsunami

victims in Japan, and the whole thing was a dramatic instrumental with some

background vocals. Since I really liked the song (and instrumentals are easier to work with in terms of choreography), I decided I could fabricate an exceptional, lyrical dance to it.

In my basement, I had multiple costumes I used to wear when I was little for recitals, and I liked to dance to my company's performance DVDs in those costumes. On my rack full of costumes, there was a red cape that I wore for an improv solo in my kindergarten talent show. It was pretty big on me then, so it fit perfectly when I put it on for "Heart." To finish my costume off, I chose a white top and skirt. We thought the red color was a nice representation for the victims and the white represented the peace they so desperately longed for.

Throughout the choreographing process, I made sure my chosen dance moves went along with the storyline we made perfectly. The dance ended up telling the story of a young girl whose family and friends passed away during the tsunami, and she expressed her feelings about it through dancing. At the end of the number, she visits her family's graves and leaves flowers by them to set the appropriate mood for the dance.

When we finished recording the whole thing, my legs felt like noodles, my chest was tight from all my heavy, intense breathing, and I was burning up. Even though I hated the tight, burning feeling in my lungs, I never wanted to stop dancing —the aches, burns, and tiredness were all worth it.

~~~~~

"My legs are *killing* me."

"Well, it is the second time we've gone up to Publix today…" I laughed, not believing how ridiculous we were to make the fifteen minute walk from my house to the stripmall outside our neighborhood that many times… plus the two going *back* to my house. We were clearly crazy—getting frozen yogurt from Yogli Mogli, buying multiple bags of candy at Publix, and walking around the few shops. By the end of our excursion, I had bought a bag of Milky Ways, Sour Patch Kids, and Jen and I got a bag of Reese's, Crunch Bars, and Rolos to share. We knew we'd be on a major sugar high after we finished eating all that candy; we hoped to somehow make it last Jen's whole stay. Also, I invited two friends to come meet Jen, and we figured they'd probably snitch some as well.

When my friends came over, we went up to the stripmall *again* and sang "Let It Go" from *Frozen*. All our walking made us hot, so when we got back to my house, we swam in my pool. We wanted to play a game, so we took my two purple noodles, and Jen and I hopped on one like a seahorse while my other two friends got on the other one the same way. After getting situated, we raced across the pool and tried our hardest not to fall off. I ended up getting dunked underwater a few times, so I was thankful I wore my goggles. Jen and I can't catch ourselves when we're about to fall, either, so the added feeling of fright from that made everything even more exhilarating; it's always great to find ways to make something fun in light of our effects from TM. And, it seems like we're able to do just that a lot.

~~~~~

Because Jen and I were together, it made sense to do something book-related, so we went over to Children's Healthcare of Atlanta's (CHOA) Day Rehab program I went to after I was discharged from the hospital. CHOA's chaplain adored *5k, Ballet, and a Spinal Cord Injury*, and she thought sharing our stories and speaking about our book to the children at Day Rehab around our age would benefit them.

Walking into Day Rehab, so many memories flooded back. I remembered crying almost everyday because I was tired and didn't feel like having e-stim hooked up to my arms. I remembered being scared to do any physical activity suggested because I didn't want to hurt myself. I remembered getting frustrated with my therapists and becoming a bit short with them. But, most of all, I remembered how ecstatic I was when I graduated and gained some of my normal, eight-year-old life back that I missed so much. Brushing those memories off, I focused on the task at hand.

We spoke to four girls about TM and how we made it a positive experience. The girls enjoyed listening to us, and we were happy to sign copies of our book and give each of them one. Because we had a great time, educating and informing other teens was then added to my list of things I wanted to do more of as a result of TM.

~~~~~

While Jen was in Atlanta, she, of course, needed to visit some tourist attractions; the perfect place was the World of Coca Cola. I had been there as a little kid before, but lots of time had passed since I last visited. When we arrived, my mom, Jen, and I learned how Coke is produced and took pictures with the Coca Cola Polar Bear. The best part, which we had been eagerly awaiting the whole visit, was the enormously delicious (and sticky!) tasting-room. Different types and flavors of Coke from many countries were available to try, and most of them were sweet; however, some tasted repulsive—specifically Beverly from Italy. Some drinks, like Beverly, were so awful that Jen and I almost spat them out and gagged, but we still managed to try every single soda in the tasting room—and there were *60* different sodas. We were both pretty hyper after that.

Near the end of Jen's visit, I kept looking at the clock and wishing we had more time together. I knew I'd see her at camp that July, but that felt extremely far away, and I didn't want to wait that long. To get more time together, we stayed up as late as we could her last night, even though I had school the next day.

When morning came, I got ready for school, and my mom drove me there with Jen. My assistant came to the car to get me, and she introduced herself to Jen. Sadness took over me so quickly, so I began crying. I was mortified to be crying in front of my assistant, and I didn't want anyone at school to see me. But, I regained my composure enough to go inside and try to get through the day after hugging Jen goodbye. She texted me during social studies and asked if I was okay, and I told her I was, but I was missing her so much already. That's the thing about long distance friendships: those that are near don't appreciate the proximity, and those that are far long for it—being miles away makes a friendship stronger.

Laughter.

Jennifer

One after another, more than 20 pieces of paper slid out of the printer in Sarah Todd's playroom.

Part of me thought that what we were doing was completely ridiculous, but the rest of me figured it was okay to be a kid and do weird-but-fun things every once in awhile.

Sarah Todd had had the idea to create our own "red carpet" in her basement and dress up nicely for a "red carpet" photoshoot. It definitely wasn't something most 16-year-olds did in their free-time, but why not? I had to admit that I kind of loved dressing up and doing photoshoots.

Unfortunately, we needed one of those big-white-backgrounds-filled-with-advertisements to complete our red carpet look, and the Hammers did not happen to have one of those just lying around their house. So, we had to embark on the slightly difficult task of creating it ourselves.

After the pieces of our backdrop were done printing, we laid them on the floor and taped them together. When we were finished, it was probably as big as a medium-sized throw blanket.

"Now… How are we going to get this downstairs?" I asked ST as I turned to face her.

"Umm… I didn't really think about that," she responded, shrugging.

"Well," I said. "I guess we'll have to fold it a little bit."

So, we did. We carefully folded the backdrop into quarters, then proceeded to walk it down to the basement. On the way there, we passed by Sarah Todd's mom in the kitchen. She lifted her head and saw us, looking a little confused, but she eventually just returned her gaze to her work.

Once we got in the basement, we conveniently found a red curtain to be the carpet-part of our red carpet. We then taped the backdrop up and laid the curtain out underneath it.

We realized a little too late that the backdrop we had made was a little too short; our heads went above the top of it when we stood up.

Oh, well.

After we finished setting all of that up, we decided to run up to ST's room to get ready for our photoshoot.

The dress I had brought with me was black on the top and a black and white chevron pattern on the bottom. The one Sarah Todd picked out was a black and white striped pattern on the top and multi-colored on the bottom.

After changing, we put on necklaces and earrings before putting on a light amount of makeup. We then asked ST's mom to help us curl our hair; however, neither of us had very curlable hair, so we both ended up with light waves on the bottom.

When we were done getting ready, Sarah Todd asked her mom to take pictures of us after explaining what we were doing. She agreed, and we all headed back down to the basement.

As soon as we stood on our "carpet" and her mom had her phone camera pointing at us, ST struck a dramatic pose. Mrs. Hammer and I laughed as she continued striking sassy, diva-like poses.

When some of the craziness was out of her system, we came up with a bunch of cute poses and got a good amount of nice-looking pictures.

"This was a weird idea I had. But it was so fun," Sarah Todd concluded when we finished.

~~~~~

There was never a dull moment when I was with ST. One day, we're creating our own fake red carpet. The next, we're randomly drawing on the driveway with chalk. My friends and I used to cover our driveways in chalk drawings all the time when we were little, but I couldn't remember the last time I'd played with it. It had probably been an incredibly long time.

"I made hopscotch!" Sarah Todd announced, pointing at what she had just drawn. I stood up and brushed my chalky hands on my shorts before walking over to her to see.

ST proceeded to jump on the squares, and I followed suit. Hopscotch was also something I hadn't played in many years.

"What else should we draw?" my friend asked. I just shrugged. We stood there a second, surveying her driveway, which was now covered in random drawings of flowers, people, and rainbows... And now hopscotch, too.

"I don't think there's much else to draw. I don't think there's much *room* to draw anymore, either," I responded, stating the obvious.

"Okay, well, we should just walk to Publix again, then!" Sarah Todd said. I had no idea why that was what she concluded, but the walks *were* pretty fun, even if they were a bit tiring. I was fine with walking there again.

"I mean, why not?" I responded.

So, we started on our millionth walk to Publix, talking and laughing the whole time.

~~~~~

It was the last night I was staying in Georgia; my flight left early the next morning. Sarah Todd and I tried to stuff as many good times into that day as we could, but we'd already managed to cross off pretty much everything that was on the list of "Things To Do At ST's House," which we had created well before I had gotten there. So, we had nothing to do, but were anxious to do *something*; we didn't want to regret wasting that time later on.

"Let's look in my closet. Maybe there's something in there," Sarah Todd said after we had been sitting on her bed for a few minutes. Both of us stood up, not having any better ideas, and walked into her closet.

"This is mostly clothes," I said after studying the area for a second.

"Yeah, but... Wait! Up there!" ST said, pointing to a high shelf above some of her clothes. I looked in the direction of her finger and saw two cubes, one red and one pink.

".... Jack-in-the-Boxes?" I asked her questioningly. She nodded with enthusiasm.

"Why not? They've been sitting in my closet since I was a toddler. I don't remember what they're like."

I couldn't think of anything better to do, so I reached up to grab them off the shelf. I took the red one down first, which I realized was decorated with *Curious George*. After handing it to ST, I grabbed the pink one, which was decorated with bears wearing tutus.

When I walked out of the closet, I saw that Sarah Todd was already turning the handle on the *Curious George* box. The classic "Pop Goes the Weasel" tune came out of it when she did. As soon as I sat beside her, the lid flipped open and a little monkey sprung out.

"AH!" ST screamed, falling back dramatically. Admittedly, I jumped a little bit, too, even though I'd seen it coming. Sarah Todd sat back up, and we looked at each other for a second before cracking up.

"That was ludicrous. This is a toy for three-year-olds, and it scared us," she said, still laughing.

We decided to try the pink jack-in-the-box next. As soon as we started turning the handle, we realized that the song was not the expected "Pop Goes the Weasel." It was something else, so we had no idea when to expect the bear to pop out.

POP

"AHH!"

We both jumped two feet in the air. The end of that song seemed to be very sudden, so the toy animal popped out much more unexpectedly than in the *Curious George* one. Once again, we erupted in a fit of giggles at the sheer ridiculousness of the situation and our reactions.

As crazy as the idea was, we had a good time, and it wasn't a bad way to spend some of my last hours in Georgia.

Anticipation.

Sarah Todd

At CCK in 2013, Jen really wanted me to perfect my favorite dance we recorded and perform it in the camp's talent show. However, I didn't think I had just the right dance to perform, and I wanted an outstanding one to share with the audience if I participated in the talent show; plus, I didn't have a suitable costume to wear onstage since the ones I'd brought were casual clothes.

Because I didn't perform the year before, I decided I would choreograph my dance to "Falling Slowly," which I had been planning to do for a few months, and perform it in 2014. Jen and I wrote a storyline for the dance, and it ended up being about a homeless girl trying to find a home and a loving family.

The talent show served as the perfect motivation for me to make my dance spectacular, and I got more and more excited about it as I played the song and improvised like I did with Jen in March. I had to take breaks after every full play of the song, and each time I rested, I went over the parts from the improv I wanted to keep in the dance. After finishing my improv, I included the moves I liked in the first 30 seconds of the song and made sure I had them memorized. I listened for any major beat changes in the song, because those are usually good points to start including dance moves that express the story I wanted the audience to perceive.

I never wanted to overdo anything, but it's difficult to convince myself to stop doing my new dance repeatedly. That was, until I attempted adding a neck dip, which is a slow, graceful leaning-back of the neck. Usually, I leaned my neck back slightly so I wouldn't hurt my weak muscles, but this time, I lost control. When I attempted to lift my neck back up straight, I couldn't do it. Panicking, I thought fast, trying not to get hurt. The only feasible solution seemed to be to lie down so that I could gain control of my neck once again. After successfully and safely lying on the ground, I lay there for a few minutes, rather scared to pursue standing up.

In general, I was very optimistic, but understandably, my temporarily pessimistic mind immediately ventured to the worst, formulating the exceedingly improbable theory that I was going to be attacked with TM once more. Since TM, every minor backache, headache, and muscle ache terrified me, even though I constantly reminded myself that I was okay and wouldn't become more paralyzed than I already was. I shoved the haunting, false thoughts away, though, and convinced myself to pull my body up slowly.

Because of this incident, I definitely knew I needed to rest, which disappointed me since I was having fun. Resting didn't stop my active mind from roaming some more, however, and I ended up wondering what would've happened if TM struck me in the middle of a performance. Would I have kept going with my headache but stopped when my arms went limp? Would I have run off the stage because my headache was excruciating? Would someone have come onstage and carried me off? The scenarios made me cringe, and I realized then that I needed to prohibit my imagination from running amok.

In all, I spent close to two hours choreographing the dance, making sure I remembered it, and resting my neck. I knew Jen, always the supportive friend, was eager to see it, so I recorded it and texted it to her after I was finished, waiting for her reaction—she'd surely love it. Of course, she thought I did an amazing job choreographing the dance, and she couldn't wait to see me perform it live, onstage. My first performance after getting TM was going to be my first solo performance ever; being able to dance was something I had learned to cherish—working arms or not.

Dedication.

Jennifer

My friends and I had been training for the half marathon all spring. Now, June 7th was finally approaching, and I was about to run the longest race of my life—*by far*.

I was very, very nervous. I knew that TM caused me to have good days and bad days; sometimes, the bad flares were so bad I could barely get out of bed. My pain and fatigue had been starting to flare a lot more frequently lately for some reason, which made it even scarier. All I could do in preparation for the race was rest a *lot* the day before—like all day—and hope with every fiber of my being that my body would decide that June 7th, 2014 was going to be a good day.

I had to wake up incredibly early that morning so we could get to the city well before the race started, and when I did, it seemed like my luck was holding; I felt okay.

Because it was so early, traffic wasn't too terrible, so before I knew it, we were in the city. I nervously chewed on my protein bar and took alternating sips of Gatorade and water. I wasn't hungry at all—in fact, I was usually nauseous in the morning—but I knew that I needed the fuel and hydration. The fact that I was a little out of my comfort zone made me a bit anxious; I knew exactly how much food and water I needed for a three-mile cross country race, but I had no idea what was best for my body before 13.1 miles. Everything about this experience was foreign and new, and like most new things, it was simultaneously exciting and terrifying.

Before I joined the crowd of people near the starting line, my mom reminded me that going fast wasn't what mattered—the experience was. Crossing the finish line was a big enough accomplishment.

I knew that, but it was easy to forget. Hearing her say it made me feel better.

I took a deep breath, then joined my friends, Grace and Sara, in the huge group of people who we thought best matched our pace. My mom, who was also running this race (though it was by no means her first half marathon), disappeared into a different group of people.

"Are you ready?" Sara asked. The three of us looked at each other, all of us clad in running clothes and pouches that held mini water bottles and energy gels. We kind of shrugged and nodded at the same time in response, clearly not sure of whether or not we were really ready for this thing.

Before I knew it, the race was starting. I didn't feel ready at all, but I knew I had to be.

No backing out now.

We moved slowly at first, the sea of people slowly inching its way to the starting line. The time it took for everyone to get to the starting line wasn't quite long enough for me to have time to collect myself, though Soon enough, we were at the start.

The start of the half marathon felt way more relaxed than most races I had run in. Cross country races, for example, were very fast and chaotic as soon as they started. For this, we all immediately fell into a nice jogging-pace.

Unfortunately, my legs decided to hurt a lot sooner than I was hoping they would. Not that I was all that surprised; running often caused almost every type of pain out there to hit my legs and even sometimes the rest of my body, too.

Whenever I ran after TM, it felt like I was running on open flames each time my feet hit the ground, and my legs ached and stung so badly, it was as if someone was hitting them repeatedly with hammers. Random stabbing and shooting pains would often run up and down my body as well.

This race, unfortunately, proved to be no exception. After only a couple miles, everything was hurting.

But I'd known going into this that unless some huge miracle was going to happen, my body was going to try to turn against me. And I could push through it; after all, I had been practicing pushing through this stuff for a couple years.

"Longest race of my life" was right. Just maybe not in the same way I had originally thought that phrase to mean.

~~~~~

By the time I could see the finish line, I was barely running anymore. Grace and I had been running together the entire time, and due to a bunch of painful blisters covering the bottoms of her feet, she had needed to take a lot more breaks than originally planned. It was definitely a lot more breaks than I would've liked since the large amount of starting and stopping aggravated my nerve pain even more, for whatever reason.

By now, my legs were dragging immensely; I could barely pick them up to take the next step each time. But I was almost there; the finish line was in sight, and I knew that it was just one foot after another before I'd be done.

Although my legs were rubbery, I knew I'd severely regret not sprinting to the finish. I always did that at the end of every race. Even on practice runs, I liked to sprint the last few seconds; it always made the run feel complete.

I was pretty sure I wouldn't be able to sprint full-out during this one, but I knew I could at least try to speed up a lot. So, I did just that, waving at Grace before I did.

I probably went from a 20 minute-per-mile pace to an eight-minute-per-mile pace, but at this point, it felt like a sprint. Reaching the finish line took no time at all, and when I crossed it, it took all of the effort and energy I had left in me to not let myself collapse. I had thought that my legs hurt badly when I was running, but it was nothing compared to stopping completely; a huge wave of indescribable pain washed over them and began pulsating through my entire body. It was one of the worst times they'd ever hurt in my life, and they also felt like they were completely made out of Jell-O. I couldn't wait to go home and sleep for two weeks.

However, as I was handed my participatory medal, I knew I was happy. I knew that the most important thing today was crossing the finish line. I didn't need an incredible time at the end of my first half marathon; I just needed to finish. That was my only goal. And it was completely worth the fact that I would barely be able to get out of bed for a long time afterwards as my body recovered.

I had just run my first half marathon at only 16 years old! Heck, I had just finished running a half marathon less than three years after being paralyzed and unable to even walk. So, yeah. Doing everything perfectly, running it in two hours or less—none of that mattered. I crossed the finish line. I was able to say that I had finished a 13.1-mile race. And I was able to say that I completed a goal I had set for myself years before, despite all the obstacles that laid in my path.

Because I completed it, I had no doubts in my mind that I had the ability to finish difficult things. Maybe, just maybe, I could run a full marathon sometime in my future. Maybe I could do a triathlon. Maybe I could do another half and improve my time significantly. Maybe I could make the varsity team in cross country next year.

The possibilities seemed endless.

Optimism.

Sarah Todd

Summer meant hanging out with friends, but more specifically, July meant hanging out with friends at CCK. Jen and I had just seen each other four months earlier, but we were never not excited to see each other. We knew this year at camp would be super special and significant with our plans of a book signing/selling and my dance, which my friends and family were eager to see.

Jen and I, of course, did our normal, fun activities such as taking millions of pictures on Photobooth and laughing at them until we thought we might pass out due to breathlessness. We also attempted to reenact our hilarious, immature videos we took at camp in 2012. They didn't turn out as good, but it was funny that we remembered almost word-for-word what we said in our old videos. In addition to my Photobooth obsession, we loved getting midnight snacks and vanilla coffee in the dining hall. All the sweets made us hyper, which made us lose sleep, but we couldn't afford to miss out on any of our time together.

~~~~~

CCK always held fun activities for the younger kids, which Jen and I usually didn't go to, but they had a carnival in the gym that we ended up going to with Abby, Bridget, and our new friend Katya. We couldn't participate in most of the games since they required arms and hands, so we mostly watched our friends do some of them. I didn't enjoy feeling left out, so Jen and Bridget suggested we try playing some games as a team. Thinking about it, I figured it could work; with our combined strength, we equaled about an average person's strength. We worked together to throw balls into the score slots, and my right arm ached by the time we finished—I was thankful we decided to work together.

One activity Jen and I could do without help that we were interested in was the fortune teller, who we knew wasn't legitimate, but we thought it would be fun. We went up to her tent, and according to her readings of our hands, she expected us to find a dollar within the next 30 days. Obviously, that never ended up occurring, but we had fun at the pretend carnival.

After the carnival, everyone hung out in the main circle at the picnic tables and chatted. Abby, Bridget, and I felt quite adventurous, and we came up with a crazy game: Bridget would sit in her wheelchair with a jump rope attached behind it, while I would sit in Abby's wheelchair and be pulled along by Bridget. We spent what felt like an hour trying to connect the two wheelchairs and cheered when we were successful. All of us knew the game clearly wasn't safe and many bad things could've happened, but it turned out that the rope wasn't strong enough to pull all the weight anyway. That was probably a good thing despite our disappointment.

~~~~~

Walking to our cabins, Jen and I talked to one of the counselors on the way. We had befriended her earlier in the dining hall and ended up talking with her for almost an hour. Enjoying her company, we decided to have her come along with us to the cabins.

When our previous conversation had died down, Courtney observed, "It looks like you two have made pretty amazing recoveries." I agreed with her 100%—I was definitely significantly better than I had been at onset about four years prior, and Jen was as well. I looked at Jen, wondering what she was thinking.

She responded, "Paralysis-wise, yeah. We've recovered quite a bit there. We both still have some arm and hand paralysis, though and lots of other issues."

"What other issues?"

I was glad she was curious and wanted to know more; her questions weren't bothering me at all. However, I did feel like she thought our problems weren't as big of a deal since we weren't in wheelchairs.

"We have pain and get tired a lot, and we have scoliosis."

Jen added, "And osteoporosis." I nodded.

"Oh, wow," Courtney said, "No one ever would've known."

~~~~~

The Messy Games had never been an activity Jen and I liked to do, so we decided to do my makeup, braid my hair messily, put my costume on, and do a photoshoot for "Adrift." Jen searched "good-looking photoshoot poses" online, and I did my favorite ballet moves in a lot of the pictures. We took some serious, sad, and happy pictures, each one being significant to the dance's storyline. In addition to all the pictures, I practiced my dance a couple times, and we recorded and kept the best one. I wasn't sure why, but every time I did my dance, I had the fear that I might forget it, and I certainly did not want that happening at the talent show.

I wanted to step on the stage, smile, have confidence, and delve into performing and entertaining that I wouldn't even think about what the next move was or what facial expression would be appropriate next. I wanted to show everyone what I could do. I wanted to listen to cheers and praises from the audience. I wanted to prove to everyone including myself that ballet was my ardor and I could perform every move with utmost grace. In my mind, I knew everything would turn out impeccable—the perfect hair, makeup, costume, and most importantly, the dance.

The next day—the day of the talent show—I knew I was right. That tiny bit of despondency I'd had immediately vanished at the first ballet step as all the others brought the confidence I knew I had. With a joyful spirit and perfect appearance, I performed my first self-choreographed solo onstage and didn't miss a beat. Going from one move to the next, I didn't even need to think; I knew I had my dance memorized. I knew every move would be perfect. I knew nothing would come to naught.

I told a story—not with my mouth, but with my feet; with every step, I added more and more to a beautiful story.

~~~~~

After hugging Jen goodbye, I watched from my car as she and her mom walked back to the dining hall. Inevitably, I'd cry when I said goodbye to Jen because I never knew when I'd see her again, and texting her just wasn't the same. Our five days at camp always went too quickly, and I always found myself wishing she was my next-door neighbor so we could see each other every day. Being the positive person I am, though, I reminded myself that I'd for sure see her within some months. I just didn't know how close that visit was, and neither did she.

Teamwork.

Jennifer

"Eating. At the table," Sarah Todd sang as she swung her phone around to record everyone. We had been at camp again for a couple days now, and the four of us—Sarah Todd, Bridget, Katya, and I—were sitting at one of the picnic tables after lunch while ST and Bridget made crazy videos. Though I'd just seen ST a few months before because I'd visited her house in March, it was still really fun to hang out with her again. Plus, I still hadn't seen my other friends in an entire year, so it was nice to spend time with them again as well.

"Eating. At the table," ST sang again, zooming in on each of us.

"I'm going to play this at your wedding," I told her, trying to maintain a serious expression as she put the phone close to my face.

"And there's me!" She squealed, ignoring me as she turned the phone around so the camera could see her face. She smiled, then turned it around to face us again.

"Eating. At the table."

~~~~~

"Do you want to try archery?" Sarah Todd asked me after breakfast the next day.

"We can try, but I don't know if we'll be very good at it," I said, laughing. Both of us had attempted archery our first year at camp, but it had been a difficult task.

"Maybe we can figure out a way. We have like... A total of two arms between us," she responded. That was true. I nodded in agreement, and we headed towards the archery area.

When we got there, both of us immediately noticed that it looked different than the last time we had tried it. There was now a wooden platform to stand on while shooting arrows at the targets, and the area was shaded with a little hut-like thing.

The two of us approached the platform where a little boy in a wheelchair was doing archery. When we saw how he was doing it, we were surprised. The bow was mounted sideways on top of the wooden rail that was at the front of the platform, so the boy didn't have to hold the heavy bow up at all; he just needed to turn it so it was in the position he wanted and pull the string back.

Sarah Todd and I looked at each other, thinking the same thing; even though it was clear that they'd adapted it this way to make it easier for wheelchair users, it would likely make it a bit more plausible for us as well.

"Would you guys like a bow?" the counselor running the activity asked us. We told her that we wanted to try it the adaptive way like the little boy was doing. She looked at us for a second, probably a little confused since we clearly weren't in wheelchairs, but she led us to an open spot.

"Do you want to go first?" I asked ST when we stood in front of the bow. She shook her head, telling me to go.

I turned the bow a bit on the mount, positioning it so it was pointing at the center of the target. Sarah Todd handed me an arrow, and I put it in the proper place, then pulled the string with my left hand while trying to steady the bow with my right. I let go, but my right hand slipped, causing the bow to move to the left. The arrow flew into the side of the target.

"Not quite in the center.... At all. You were not even close. But at least you hit it?" ST said from beside me while laughing a little bit.

"I never said I was a good aim," I responded, giggling. "Let's see if you can do better."

I stepped to the side so my friend could stand in front of the bow. She studied it for a second before I handed her an arrow.

She tried to get the arrow in the bow, but it was a little tricky, so I helped her out. She placed her left hand on the bow in an attempt to steady it, then pulled the string and let go.

But she didn't have enough strength to pull the taut string back very far, so the arrow fell straight down, landing only a few inches in front of our feet.

"Okay, wait," Sarah Todd said. "What if we try to do it together? I can steady the bow with my left hand, and you can steady it with your right on the other side. Then we can both pull the string together with our better hands!"

I thought that sounded like a great idea, so I agreed. I walked over to the right of her, and she took a couple steps to the left so there was room for me. Sarah Todd positioned the bow so it was straight, and I grabbed another arrow and set it up. I held onto the arrow and part of the string while ST grabbed onto some of the string next to it.

"Okay, count of three, and we'll let go," I said.

"One," ST started. "Two... THREE!"

We both let go and watched as the arrow flew across the little field and landed near the center of the bulls-eye.

~~~~~

Every day after lunch at CCK is the designated "siesta" time. Usually my friends and I just hung out in the gym or one of our lodges, but today was different; the camp coordinators were allowing ST and I to sign and sell copies of *5k, Ballet, and a Spinal Cord Injury* in the dining hall. Though it was still technically "siesta time" for everyone else, they were all notified of our signing and encouraged to come.

"I'm excited! I love signing books. I hope people buy some," Sarah Todd said, practically jumping up and down while we watched a couple counselors set a table up in the middle of the room.

The counselors placed two chairs in front of the table before walking away. ST's mom walked in then, carrying a cardboard box filled with books. She placed the box under the table and helped us set our display out on the top of the table.

Sarah Todd and I sat down at the table—both wearing our turquoise-colored *5k, Ballet, and a Spinal Cord Injury* t-shirts—and waited for people to come in.

Our friend Katya walked into the dining hall first, carrying one of her "Katya Strong" t-shirts and her copy of our book. When she approached our table, she asked us to sign both the shirt and the book. Signing a shirt was unexpected, of course, but we happily complied. After we returned the signed items to her, Katya pulled a chair up near our table and kept us company for a while.

After that, some other people came into the dining hall every few minutes. Some already had books that they'd previously bought online and just wanted to get them signed, but most of them bought copies from us there.

Unfortunately, "siesta-time" had to end eventually and, consequently, so did our signing.

"That was really fun! I'm glad the camp let us set it up!" Sarah Todd said as we were leaving the dining hall to go to the next activity on our agenda. I smiled, nodding in agreement.

"Abby and I are having an election! Do you vote for me?" Bridget pleaded a random camper. The kid nodded, and Bridget cheered, pumping her fists in the air.

"YES! Thank you! ABBY! I GOT ANOTHER VOTE! I'M WINNING!"

"Well, I got two more! That's 14. We're tied again," Abby shouted from across the field. Bridget groaned, throwing her head back.

"No! I'm going to ask some more people," she announced before wheeling in the opposite direction. Sarah Todd and I sat at one of the picnic tables, laughing as we watched the scene unfold.

Earlier that day, ST and I had randomly taken "campaign videos" of both Bridget and Abby. We asked what they would do to better our country if they ran for president. The two girls took it further, though, and began competing to see who could get the most "votes."

"Do you vote for me or Bridget?" Abby asked a lady sitting near ST and me.

"Sorry, I already told Bridget that she has my vote. She can be very persuasive," the lady said apologetically. Abby sighed dramatically and moved on to the next person.

"I think I'm supposed to be like her campaign manager or something. I should go help her," Sarah Todd said to me before leaving our table, presumably to persuade people to "vote" for Abby. I was technically supposed to be on Bridget's "side" while ST was on Abby's, but it didn't look like Bridget needed much assistance. Anyway, going up to random people wasn't really my thing.

Eventually, the sky darkened, and counselors started setting up a fire-pit and s'mores ingredients as well as a big projector that was going to project *Monsters University* on the side of a building for us to watch outside. They set up a bunch of chairs and blankets on the lawn as well, and I left my spot at the picnic table to save some seats for my friends.

Right as I thought I was going to have to get up and search for them, I saw Bridget, Abby, and Sarah Todd heading over to where I was sitting.

"I think I won!" Bridget announced triumphantly.

~~~~~

Every year, the last day of camp held one of the biggest highlights of the week: the talent show. This year, Sarah Todd was performing in it. She had been working so hard at creating and perfecting both this dance specifically and her dance techniques in general.

As I watched my friend perform onstage, I couldn't help but be immensely proud of her. I had watched so many of her dances over the last two years and knew just how far she'd come.

I couldn't wait to see what the future would bring.

Passion.

Sarah Todd

786 VIEWS

I looked at the view count on my "Adrift" dance video uploaded to YouTube, and I couldn't believe it. Loads of people had seen my dance, my dance that I was so proud of, and I couldn't be happier. Watching the video for the first time, I was a bit emotional because everything was how I wanted it to look—the costume, hair and makeup, choreography, and performance—and I honestly couldn't believe I had actually done it all. After discontinuing classes at ADT, I never thought I'd get up on a real stage and do what I love most again—let alone an extremely powerful self-choreographed solo.

When I first went back to my ballet classes, I thought everything would go right back to normal and I'd perform in all my shows once again. Obviously, none of that worked out the way I hoped, but I have a new, eminent alternative that I grew fond of quickly because my original plan didn't work out as I'd expected.

Afterall, dancers dance with their heart, mind, and soul—when I pas de chat, my arms aren't in first position; when I jeté, my arms aren't in arabesque; when I pirouette, my arms aren't in first position, but my heart, mind, and soul are there through every determined move and beat.

With determination, it is possible to block out the negative things and enjoy the positive ones, despite the cons. Most importantly, it is possible to dance through everything pernicious.

Steadfastness.

Jennifer

When I looked back on those past two years, I realized that I'd come much further than it seemed. After all, I went from being an almost-freshman running ten-minute miles to a 16-year-old running a half marathon; that was a significant amount of progress in just two years.

In 2011, when I was lying in the hospital at onset, I had fears of never running again. Though a big part of me thought that I'd be able to recover fully in no time, those fears were always subtly present in the back of my mind.

In 2012, when I ran that first timed mile in over ten minutes, I became discouraged and wasn't sure if I'd ever be able to get back to where I was before August 16th, 2011. But I pushed myself greatly, always making it to the finish line. And I excelled; each race brought improvements, even if they weren't obvious ones. It's definitely likely that I would've been faster and "better" had TM—with all the challenges it brought to every run—not been an obstacle, but still, I excelled more than I'd ever imagined when lying in that hospital bed or sulking after that ten-minute mile.

So, looking back on those two years, I had goals for the future. I had goals to run full marathons and triathlons and improve my three-mile time enough that I could go to the State cross country meet junior or senior year. And, when looking at just how much I'd done in those past two years, those goals seemed possible. I was excited to see what I'd achieve in the future.

But, of course, the future is always uncertain. And the thing about life is, you never know what it will throw at you next.

"It has never been my object to record my dreams, just the determination to realize them."

- Man Ray

Afterword

In this book, more of our stories are told from June 2012-July 2014, and unlike in *5k, Ballet, and a Spinal Cord Injury*, no big, sudden changes happened in our lives during the time it takes place. However, we are all growing and learning and changing every single day, and that is evident throughout *Determination*.

This book primarily focuses on our evolution in running and dancing. One of the biggest themes in *5k, Ballet* was the fight and journey to run and dance again. However, though we were ecstatic to get back to doing our favorite things, that was just the beginning; we still had a lot ahead of us, including both failures and successes, and we hope that this book does an excellent job of conveying that.

In the beginning of *Determination*, Sarah Todd talked about dancing to her old dance company's videos and how much she missed dancing in those shows. Though she regained the ability to dance, *just* dancing to those videos wasn't quite enough. This book went through some of ST's struggles and failures, including when she tried to dance with a yardstick and tried to make her arms look the way she wanted them to. She went through a journey of trying new things when it came to dancing, eventually leading her to her big success: choreographing and performing "Adrift" onstage in front of everyone at the Center for Courageous Kids. Performing for people again, as well as teaching herself to choreograph—something she never did before TM—fulfilled Sarah Todd more than she thought possible when wistfully watching and dancing to her old company's videos in 2012.

As for Jen, she started out by being barely able to run in cross country camp in 2012. She progressed to a ten-minute mile, then to a seven-minute mile. Jen had some discouraging races, ones where she was slow or TM caused a lot of obstacles; however, she ran a three-mile race in 22:45, then 21:45 a year later, then crossed the finish line of a half marathon. This evolution was gradual, for the most part, and the discouraging races often overshadowed the good ones in her mind, but her success ended up fulfilling her in ways she never thought possible in the beginning.

Of course, this book was not strictly about our progress in our sports. It also showed the evolution in friendship, both between the two of us and our other TM friends. It showed more of the normal chronic illness/disability struggles as well—from the everyday challenges that come from having Transverse Myelitis to huge doctor appointments in different states. Through all of these different themes, *Determination* illustrates how we matured and grew in many aspects of our lives from June 2012 to July 2014.

Before every chapter in this book was a powerful word: courage, performance, aspiration, stubbornness, energy, joy, empathy, support, encouragement, diligence, strength, willpower, dependability, endurance, decision, stamina, effort, fortitude, patience, guidance, inspiration, gratefulness, enjoyment, commitment, confidence, perseverance, wisdom, motivation, dreams, goals, spirit, laughter, anticipation, dedication, optimism, teamwork, passion, and steadfastness.

All of these are qualities that we possessed during the events throughout this book as we matured and evolved in so many different ways.

Through determination, we were able to possess all the qualities each of those words display.

If we weren't determined, neither of us would have dreams, goals, patience, strength, optimism, dedication, etc., and neither of us would've accomplished all we have.

Acknowledgments

We'd like to thank everyone who helped us make our book be the absolute best it could be, as well as our friends, family, and everyone else who has supported us.

This book took a long time to write; the first two and a half years or so were spent writing the first half of the book while the second half was written in about a month. We gave ourselves a deadline and clearly, we both work best under pressure. See? With ***determination***, a book can be written in very little time!

Each of us thanks the other for their encouragement and cooperation throughout the writing process—we can both be stubborn, but we dealt with each other and produced a masterpiece! And we both made it out alive. Somehow.

Thanks to you, too, for reading!

About The Authors

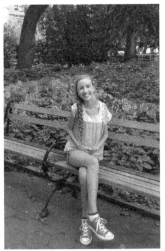

Sarah Todd Hammer is 14 years old and in ninth grade. She has had Transverse Myelitis for six years. She lives in Atlanta, Georgia with her mom, dad, two older brothers, dog, and fish. Sarah Todd's favorite hobbies are dancing, choreographing, singing, acting, and writing. She has choreographed many dances, including ones to the songs "Falling Slowly" and "Therapy." Sarah Todd's absolute favorite band is One Direction. She also greatly admires and loves the musical *Hamilton*, and she loves singing every song from the show. Sarah Todd aspires to be a neurologist or psychologist.

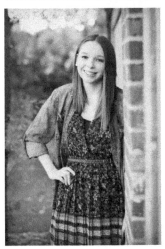

Jennifer Starzec is 18 years old and in her freshman year in college. She has had Transverse Myelitis for five years. She lives near Chicago, Illinois with her mom, dad, four younger brothers, younger sister, dog, and three cats. Jen's favorite hobbies are singing, reading, and writing. Recently, she has gotten into swimming, as well. She loves listening to (and belting) songs from musicals such as *Les Miserables*, *Hamilton*, and *Phantom of the Opera*. Jen aspires to be a physician assistant or audiologist.